Judy Bailey ONZM is a writer and former broadcaster living in Auckland. She fronted primetime news for 26 years, becoming one of the most recognised faces in New Zealand. On leaving TVNZ, she wrote a bestselling memoir, *My Own Words*. She also co-presented Māori Television's ANZAC Day programme for many years. She is a founding member and patron of Brainwave Trust Aotearoa, and a patron of organisations including the National Collective of Women's Refuges, Hospice North Shore, Skylight Trust, the Grief Centre and the Muscular Dystrophy Association. She is married to producer and director Chris Bailey, with whom she has three children and seven grandchildren.

T0359418

JUDY BAILEY

Evolving

HarperCollins*Publishers*

HarperCollins*Publishers*
Australia • Brazil • Canada • France • Germany • Holland • India
Italy • Japan • Mexico • New Zealand • Poland • Spain • Sweden
Switzerland • United Kingdom • United States of America

First published in 2024
by HarperCollins*Publishers* (New Zealand) Limited
Unit D1, 63 Apollo Drive, Rosedale, Auckland 0632, New Zealand
harpercollins.co.nz

A catalogue record for this book is available from the National Library of New Zealand

ISBN 978 1 7755 4204 9 (pbk)
ISBN 978 1 7754 9235 1 (ebook)

Cover design by Hazel Lam, HarperCollins Design Studio
Cover image by Are Media/Robert Trathen
Quote on p. 93: *From Learning to Speak Alzheimer's* by Joanne Koenig Coste. Copyright © 2003
by Joanne Koenig Coste. Used by permission of HarperCollins Publishers.
Epigraph on p. 159: From *The World According to Mister Rogers* by Fred Rogers, copyright
© 2003. Reprinted by permission of Hachette Books, an imprint of Hachette Book Group, Inc.
Typeset in Minion Pro by Kelli Lonergan
Printed and bound in Australia by McPherson's Printing Group

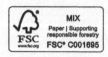

MIX
Paper | Supporting
responsible forestry
FSC
www.fsc.org FSC® C001695

For Chris.

It has been a joy to evolve with you these past 50 years.

CONTENTS

Author's note

This book contains general information in relation to your physical and financial well-being, but it does not take into account individual circumstances and is not intended as a substitute for professional advice. Always consult with a qualified medical expert for health decisions, and your lawyer or accountant for legal and financial advice.

PROLOGUE

*'Ageing is not a problem to be fixed or a disease to
be cured. It is a natural, powerful, lifelong process
that unites us all.'*

—Ashton Applewhite, 'Let's end ageism', TED Talk

The other day, my friend Stella, an effervescent 70-year-old, asked me, 'What is your definition of "old"?'

I struggled to come up with an answer.

'Pick an age,' she encouraged.

'Well ... maybe 90?' I offered.

'So, 20 years older than we are, then?' she said.

We laughed about it, because it's so true, isn't it? Particularly as we pass middle age. In a way, it really is as good a definition of 'old' as any: 20 years older than you are at any given moment!

As I write this now, I definitely don't *feel* old. A little more grown-up than I once was, perhaps, but not necessarily old. Even at 94 my mum, bless her, would often tell me she still felt '24 inside', and I know what she meant. On the inside, she *was* essentially still the same person. A lifetime of experiences had shaped her, and outwardly she'd changed, but she was still Dinny Morrison. She still had the same sense of humour, the same love of life and family, the same anxieties, the same basic needs. It didn't really make much difference whether she was 94 or 24.

Or rather it *shouldn't* have made much difference. But, now that I'm into my seventies, I know it does make a difference. I find my advancing age inescapable. Gloomy? No. That is precisely what I *don't* want to be about the inevitability of age. Growing older is a blessing, one so many don't get to experience. After all, I hope to have 20 or even 30 good summers left in me and I don't want to waste them!

However, as those of us unceremoniously lumped into the amorphous category of 'old' know all too well, there's a lot more to ageing than how you feel on the inside. There are also all the ways things on the outside are changing – and I'm not just talking about your looks. Yes, there are the signs you spot when you look in the mirror. I like to put a positive spin on these ones. 'I'll never look better,' I think, as I peer into the magnifying mirror in the bathroom. Optimistic, and also true … The wrinkles will eventually win! And that mirror, of course, turns every one of them into a giant chasm. Mind you, I couldn't do without it, or I'd end up wearing my lipstick in my eyebrows.

But there are other changes, too. Ones that have to do with the way you're seen by the world, the way you're treated. Ones that started popping up for me back when I was in my early fifties. I was still working as a news anchor then, and ahead of the bulletin one night I was reviewing a story about an 'elderly' woman who had been attacked. 'How old was she, exactly?' I asked the young reporter.

'Oh, about 50,' came the breezy reply.

How bloody depressing! I'd apparently skipped middle age and gone straight to 'elderly' without even realising it.

Yes, the 'old' thing sneaks up on you when you least expect it. All of a sudden, pharmacists and supermarket staff are speaking very slowly and loudly to you, you get the senior discount without people checking first, police officers and doctors really do start to look like children, and everyone assumes you don't understand technology. And then the day comes when a shop assistant decides to call you 'dear'. This one also started happening to me in my fifties. These assistants no doubt mean well, but their 'dear' I certainly am not! Honestly, it sets my teeth on edge and makes me want to reach over the counter and throttle them. Am I overreacting? If so, I'm not the only one. 'When people in grocery stores call me "dear",' 80-year-old Tess, one of the many older people I interviewed for this book, told me, 'I feel like picking them up by the collar and letting them dangle. I just reply, "Thank you, *sweetie*."'

And don't even mention the R-word. That one started creeping into conversations when I left TVNZ at the age of 54. 'So,' everyone kept asking, 'how are you finding retirement?'

'I'm not retired,' I would reply. 'I'm just not working in television anymore.'

What was it about the word 'retire' that I so loathed? Probably that it made me feel as though, because I wasn't 'on air' anymore,

I didn't have anything to offer. I felt surplus to requirements, dismissed. Not paid, therefore not productive. Honestly, I still don't much like the word. Just hearing it makes me feel instantly tired and less-than. Look it up in the dictionary and you'll see it means to withdraw, retreat, call it a day, go to bed. Sometimes when I hear it, I want to say, 'OK … If that's what you think, I'll hit the sack and pull the covers over my head.'

Again, I'm not the only one. 'I have never liked the word "retirement",' Serena Williams told *Vogue*, when she announced she was stepping away from professional tennis in late 2022. 'I've been thinking of this as a transition … Maybe the best word to describe what I'm up to is *evolution*. I'm here to tell you that I'm evolving away from tennis, toward other things that are important to me.'

I love that. Indeed, 'evolving' is what we're all doing, all the time. We move from one stage of life into another, just as the butterfly emerges from the chrysalis. Ageing is no different. Our later years should be some of our best – the stats tell us our eighties are the happiest years of our lives, for those of us lucky enough to make it that far. Yet so many of us dread older age. Why?

The ageing process is a minefield. It's sobering, getting old. You start to sense your own mortality. Life suddenly telescopes. You begin to think seriously about the time you have left. It can be a period of great uncertainty. Many of us grapple with the very real worries of losing our lifelong partners, finding ourselves alone, experiencing physical and mental decline, lacking a sense of purpose, becoming invisible. I've lost count of the number of people who've told me they feel 'invisible' because of their age –

according to New Zealand's Office for Seniors/Te Tari Kaumātua, it's 20 per cent of people over 50. And it seems to happen especially in shops. 'You can be standing there for ages at the counter and no one seems interested in helping you,' 73-year-old interviewee Patti told me. 'I can only imagine the shop assistants are short-sighted. If only they realised the amount of disposable income going begging!'

And you do begin to feel just that little bit vulnerable. That vulnerability comes, I think, from what we're told about ageing. So much of it is negative: we'll be frail, dependent, impoverished. A drain on the health system, on society. A burden. This is ageism, and it's just as toxic as every other –ism out there. It's the idea that people become somehow inferior just because of the number of years they've lived.

In 2020, the Centre for Better Ageing in the UK released a report that noted in particular how 'women's ageing is often seen more negatively than men's'. Although older women might be stereotyped as supposedly being nice things like moral, polite and empathetic, we're simultaneously deemed less competent. We are treated with a general lack of respect. Society tends to display a kind of benign indifference towards us. Perhaps that explains why Tess and I so despise being called 'dear'.

Gerontologist Dame Peggy Koopman-Boyden says a lot of older people assume they'll be given respect, but they also have to earn it. 'Never refuse an offer of help from a younger person without saying, "Thank you". Be respectful yourself; if you're on the bus standing, say "Excuse me, would you please give me your seat? I'm a bit wobbly."'

Ageism cuts both ways – it can also be directed at people for being 'too young' – but when it's targeted at older people it results in people fearing getting old. It causes us to be ashamed of our age, rather than proud of and grateful for it. But it doesn't have to be this way.

We need to change the way we think about old age. Instead of fearing the inevitable, let's start looking forward to the evolution.

* * *

Why do we slap the 'old' label on anyone over 50? It doesn't make any sense. It's an incredibly limiting thing to do to such an enormous and diverse group of people. After all, we don't lump five-year-olds in with 30-year-olds. So why do it to older people?

We are not one gigantic, homogenous mass. We are individuals, each with our own life experience to call on, with our own capabilities and talents and quirks. Some of us are in great health, others not so much. Some of us might be heading out paddleboarding every day into our nineties, while others of us are content to sit with a book. We are people. We each want different things. Just like everyone else!

By 2036, New Zealanders over 65 are predicted to spend $50 billion dollars in the local economy per year. We will likely be contributing $25 billion to the economy in unpaid voluntary work. We will be paying around $13 billion in tax. We are, it would seem, of great economic value to this country, yet we are being overlooked and misrepresented. Products developed for us focus primarily on disability, poor health or the negative signs of ageing: dentures, diapers, colour for greying hair, creams for sagging skin ... There's not a lot out there for people over 65 who see themselves as fit and healthy.

Today, people are living longer than ever before. The average life expectancy in New Zealand is now 80 for males, 83.5 for females. (Now there's a salutary thought: if this was a hundred years ago, it's unlikely that I would even be here to write this!) And, while health conditions and medical prescriptions can certainly increase with age, thanks to the wonders of medical science many of us will continue to live productive lives into ripe old age. It's heartening to know that, in fact, only a relatively small proportion of us (around 10 per cent) will eventually need full-time care. According to researchers from Harvard, while older people might find themselves living with one (or more) age-related diseases, they can still lead active, interesting lives. Life goes on, as does the ability to enjoy it.

Time's a marchin', as they say. Seize the day! To age is a privilege, after all.

We older generations have a wealth of experience and knowledge to share. What's more, we have the time to share it. Legendary American architect Frank Lloyd Wright started designing New York's Solomon R. Guggenheim Museum when he was 76, and was still working on it when he died at 91. (It opened six months after his death in 1959.) Spanish cellist Pablo Casals kept practising his music into his nineties, because he was still, in his words, 'making progress'. Nancy Pelosi, the first woman to ever hold the office of Speaker of the US House of Representatives, has only relatively recently stepped down from the role at the age of 83. She continues her political work, fighting for equality and blazing a trail for women in US politics. And, in 2021, at the age of 89, physicist Manfred Steiner received his PhD from Brown University in the US. When asked why he decided to pursue higher education in his retirement, he answered, 'If you have a dream, follow it … It is important not to waste your older days. There is a lot of brainpower in older people and I think it can be of enormous benefit to younger generations. Older people have experience and many times history repeats itself.'

'Old age is like a minefield,' said American psychiatrist and Harvard professor George Vaillant. 'If you see footprints leading to the other side … step in them.' Vaillant knew what he was talking about – he was, for three decades, the director of the lauded Harvard Study of Adult Development.

'Why step in other's footprints?' you might ask. 'Why not blaze a trail of your own?'

Well, while I do like the idea of blazing a trail into old age, I also believe we can learn so much from those who've gone before. If I am indeed traversing a minefield, I'd be mad not to step in others' footprints. I'd also be wise to clear some mines for those who come after me.

Which brings me to this book. In these pages, you'll join me on my personal journey through ageing. You'll read about my hopes and fears, about the things that bring me joy and contentment. I suspect you'll be facing and feeling some similar things. My aim? To learn all I can about ageing as happily and healthily as possible, and share what I learn with you.

My hope is that, whatever your situation or perspective, you will find something in here that inspires you.

PART 1

Health

1

YOUR WHOLE BEING
Age inside and out

'The way we choose to live life matters.'
—Gary Fraser, Adventist Health Studies

I recently attended the reunion of my 1970 journalism class. We're all in our seventies now, and hadn't seen each other for more than 50 years, but the moment we were back together the years melted away. We were soon enjoying each other's company just the way we did in our early twenties. Still just as actively engaged in and curious about life, still keen to dance the night away ...

We took this as completely normal, but it seemed to come as a surprise to the people running the vineyard where the reunion took place.

'You're all so alive,' the receptionist marvelled, seeing how much fun we were having.

I'm not sure quite what they expected. Perhaps that we should have been tucked up with our Zimmer frames, out of harm's way?!

There is a view out there that older people are different from other human beings, not subject to the same desires, concerns and fears. Not able to do the same things we might have once enjoyed. At worst, we're overlooked entirely; at best, relegated to the 'wise-but-boring' category. Back in the 1970s, when I was just starting out as a reporter on the Christchurch regional news show *The South Tonight*, I had an older colleague who was in her late fifties. I was utterly in awe of Helen Holmes. She was tall, elegant and grey-haired, a thoroughly experienced and capable journalist, with a searingly dry wit. In my mind, she was the epitome of dignity, someone who exuded gravitas in every way. So imagine my surprise the day I came to work to see her whip off all her clothes and sit stark naked behind her typewriter (fortunately slightly bulkier than today's computers!) to deliver a piece to camera about National Nudists Day. Well, that blew all my preconceptions out of the water! She didn't have a stuffy bone in her body.

In youth's defence, we can be our own worst enemies as we age, groaning when we get up from the sofa or out of the car. 'I'm having a senior moment,' we say, or 'Whoops, dementia setting in!' when we lose the car keys. (Young adults lose their keys, too, but they don't beat themselves up over it.) We even give each other 'funny' birthday cards about getting old. (You know the ones: 'Happy 40th birthday! Remember to start taking daily multivitamins and fibre supplements, you old fogey!') These cards begin to come thick and fast as you hit your forties, although I have noticed I don't seem to get quite so many of them now ... Perhaps they're a little close to the bone for a 70-year-old!

It's hardly surprising that we make ageist comments about ourselves and others. Our whole lives, we've been fed a constant diet of negative images of ageing. It can be tempting to start looking back with rose-tinted glasses, to remember how things were better 'back in our day' or how much fun we 'used to have'. However, doing so really just reinforces the notion that as we age we stop enjoying things. That we become different people.

It's time to do away with these ideas about ageing. Older people are not incapable of doing things, and we are not obliged to sit quietly in the corner. We have so much to offer, and we're eager to share it. We want to be part of the world in just the same way as everyone else wants to. While we're at it, we'd also like to have a bit of fun! Especially since, as it turns out, taking a positive view of things is as good for our bodies as it is for our souls.

A state of mind

It's generally thought that our life spans are only partially determined by our genes – twins studies, for instance, have suggested genetics account for only about 30 per cent of a person's chance of surviving to 85. So what about the rest of it? No surprises here. It turns out the other crucial ingredient in how long we live is *how* we live. That's about more than just having a good diet and working out. It's also about how you choose to live, and crucially it's about the people in your life and the strength of your relationships.

We are not programmed for longevity anyway. We're programmed to procreate. Once we've done that, we can stick around to help raise the next generation … but then what? Personally, I don't even know if I want to live to be a hundred, not if it means sitting in a chair in a rest home staring at the walls. What really matters to me is living a fulfilling life. I want to be as healthy as possible so I can enjoy life for as long as possible.

While it's no fun living to an old age if you're sick and miserable, sickness doesn't per se preclude healthy ageing. We will, most of us, have to deal with some sort of ailment as we age, whether it be arthritis or trouble with the arteries, bunions or blood pressure. But the thing we get to choose is our attitude to illness, and that makes an enormous difference. To quote the Harvard Study of Adult Development's George Vaillant, 'It's OK to be ill, so long as you don't wallow in it.'

There is a school of thought that says it's unrealistic to only ever portray ageing seniors as confident and happy, but so is painting later life solely as a time of frailty and decline, of vulnerability and dependence. The latter, in my mind, simply limits people's beliefs about their own capabilities and their own future. The truth is, it's a sliding scale, and most older people will find themselves sitting nearer the vibrant end, even if they are dealing with the diseases of age. Take heart! One enormous literature review in 2020 'forcefully confirmed' that our sense of happiness and well-being – no matter where in the world we are – tends to follow a U-shaped curve. In other words, we are happiest at the beginning and end of our lives. Things are looking up!

The Newcastle 85+ study, which began in 2006, was the first stage of the biggest population-based longitudinal study of health and ageing in over-85s anywhere in the world. Led by a research team at Newcastle University in the UK and comprising a cohort of over a thousand 85-year-olds, it examined biological, clinical and psychological factors associated with healthy ageing. None of the participants had perfect medical health – they were 85, after all! – but around three quarters of them rated their health as 'good' compared with others the same age. In other words, they might have had the odd health issue, but most of them still felt pretty sprightly.

Furthermore, just because you're old, you don't have to resign yourself to remaining ill. The previous view of ageing was that the body is like a car: over time, and with repeated use, it wears out and eventually breaks down. In some ways, this is true – but this breakdown is not as inevitable as we think. In fact, the body is capable of immense repair, although as we get older that ability to repair decreases, particularly if the body is suffering cellular damage caused by inflammation, stress, bad nutrition or other environmental factors. It's largely a matter of taking care of what you've got. University of Auckland professor Ngaire Kerse, who holds the Joyce Cook Chair in Ageing Well, is firmly of the belief that even 89-year-olds can recover from illness or injury. 'Society should let them and expect them to recover,' she says. 'You can get better.'

So, if you've ever heard that life is a downward spiral from 85, consign those thoughts to the bin!

Live well (like a Blue Zoner!)

Back in the early 2000s, demographic researchers Gianni Pes and Michel Poulain coined the term 'Blue Zones', since also used by author Dan Buettner, to describe the places in the world where they believe people are living longer, healthier, happier lives than anywhere else. The trio zeroed in on five of these Blue Zones: Okinawa, Japan; Sardinia, Italy; Nicoya, Costa Rica; Ikaria, Greece; and Loma Linda, California, US.

Poulain and Pes were both studying longevity in Sardinia when they first came up with this Blue Zones idea. Their study centred on the Sardinian highlands, and they identified Sardinia as the region of the world with the highest concentration of male centenarians. Here, people weren't just living longer; they were living well. These centenarians were still chopping wood, tending their flocks, riding their motorbikes and enjoying the company of others at the local bar. What's more, they were celebrated and played an active role within their families. Researchers have suggested this enhances an older person's sense of self-worth, which in turn gives them an extra four to six years of life expectancy.

In Okinawa, another Blue Zone, people eat a diet rich in plants, with little meat or fish. They also practise hara hachi bu, a Confucian teaching that instructs people to eat until they are 80 per cent full. Really difficult if you were raised, as I was, to eat everything on your plate! Especially as portions seem to keep getting bigger and bigger ... But the Okinawans have a way round that, traditionally using smaller plates, which restrict portion size.

There is no word for retirement in Okinawa. Instead, people talk about ikigai, the reason for which you wake up in the morning. And, similarly to the Sardinians, that reason often comes from involvement in the family, with grandparents often helping to raise grandchildren. As Buettner noted in a piece published in the *American Journal of Lifestyle Medicine*, one centenarian he spoke to in Okinawa described holding her great-great-great-grandchild as being like 'jumping into heaven'. How lovely is that?

And then there's moai, the tradition of forming strong social networks. In Okinawa, Buettner reported, children are put into moai groups at age five and continue to meet regularly for a common purpose throughout their lives. One specific moai Buettner heard of had been together for 97 years, and the average age of the group was 102. 'They meet every day to drink sake and gossip,' he wrote. This backs up the findings of multiple research projects around the world, which show socialising is a profoundly protective factor in ageing well.

Another Blue Zone, Loma Linda in California, is home to a big community of Seventh Day Adventists, known for having a lower risk of certain diseases than other Americans. Many researchers have hypothesised that this is due to the Adventists' dietary and lifestyle habits, and, for over 40 years, the Loma Linda community has been the subject of a series of long-term medical research projects looking into the link between lifestyle, diet, disease and mortality. The Adventist Health Studies, as they're collectively known, have found that Adventist men are living just over seven years longer, on average, than other American men, while the women live about four years longer than average. Notable characteristics of the Adventist lifestyle include time spent outside in the fresh air, regular exercise (especially walking outside in nature) and a plant-based diet.

Heart surgeon Ellsworth Wareham is just one example of Loma Linda's long-lived Adventists. At the age of 95, he was still performing open heart surgery, and would do around 20 procedures a month. When he was interviewed three years later, he was still sharp as a tack, his balance was good and his hands were steady. His hospital wanted him to continue operating, but he wanted to spend more time with his family. Wareham's advice for happy longevity? Keep your cholesterol below 140, eat a plant-based diet, take a calm approach to the problems of life, sleep well and don't worry. ('Easier said than done!' I hear you say.) The remarkable Dr Wareham died in 2018 at the age of 104.

Yet another Loma Linda legend is Marge Jetton, who was still lifting weights and volunteering at several organisations at the age of 104. A retired nurse, she woke every morning at 4.30 to read her Bible, and reckoned her faith held her together. She walked around one and a half kilometres before breakfast, then did more than nine kilometres on her stationary bike in the afternoon. Marge died at 106. She volunteered every day and used to say, 'If you're healthy and feel valued at 100, you'll feel 70.' I want to be like Marge!

Meanwhile, in the other Blue Zones of Nicoya in Costa Rica and Ikaria in Greece, centenarians also lead active physical lives, working in the fields or walking to visit family and friends. Those in Greece also have the added benefit of thermal springs, which are said to improve circulation, help with digestion and relieve pain.

According to Buettner, there are nine characteristics the Blue Zoners have in common.

1. **They move naturally.** They live in environments that prompt them into movement without thinking. They garden, work outside and do household chores without mechanical aids. They are definitely not sitting in cars, on sofas or at desks for hours on end!

2. **They have a sense of purpose.** A reason to get up in the morning is worth seven extra years of life.

3. **They downshift.** Stress is a big contributor to inflammation in the body. Blue Zoners still experience stress, but they commonly take time out to remember their ancestors, pray and nap.

4. **They limit the amounts and times they eat.** Like the Okinawans, Blue Zoners only eat until they're 80 per cent full. They also eat their smallest meal in the late afternoon or early evening, then don't eat anything else for the rest of the day.

5. **They eat more plants than anything else.** They take 95 per cent of their calories from plants, and the rest from animal products.

6. **They enjoy wine.** Just one or two glasses a day, with food.

7. **They belong to some form of faith-based community.** According to Buettner, this appears to add as much as 14 years to life expectancy.

8. **They put family first.** Blue Zoners invest time and love in their children and other family relationships, including commitment to a life partner.
9. **They have the right tribe.** They find like-minded people to socialise with.

According to Buettner, the average American's life expectancy could increase by as much as 12 years by adopting a Blue Zone lifestyle. More importantly, though, it'd also improve the average person's quality of life. What's not to like?

It's also interesting to note that many of the above characteristics are repeated in the key factors to healthy ageing identified by the Harvard Study of Adult Development. The world's longest longitudinal study of adult development, it began in 1938 and now includes the offspring of the original participants. (This study also included Lewis Terman's study of 90 women who were born in 1910, and in the mid-1970s 500 men from the poorest neighbourhoods in inner-city Boston were also studied. So it's not just a study about privileged white men!) This study found that people with fewer than four of the following factors were three times as likely to die before age 80.

1. **No smoking.** This one's the biggie: not being a heavy smoker or stopping young vastly improves your chances of ageing healthily.
2. **Look on the bright side.** Have the mindset that makes lemonade from lemons.

3. **Don't make mountains out of molehills.** Keep things in perspective. This predicts a better quality of life in older age.

4. **Drink alcohol responsibly.** Abusing alcohol can harm relationships, work and physical health. While the jury is still out on exactly *how much* alcohol is safe to drink, most studies recommend some time during the week off alcohol altogether. On the other hand, some suggest a glass of wine with dinner could even be beneficial. Overall, I think the general message is: restrict your intake!

5. **Nurture loving relationships.** Close relationships (such as a happy marriage) with people who understand you and with whom you're relaxed provide both company and the knowledge that you've got someone there to rely on when things turn pear-shaped.

6. **Seek higher education.** Apparently there are two reasons that having a higher education plays a part in health. First, it gives you the capacity to take a long view, enabling further education and self-care. Second, education allows you to appreciate the link between your own behaviour and its consequences.

7. **Maintain a healthy weight.** According to the Adventist Health Studies, those with a BMI between 24 and 28 were the people who tended to do best from the Loma Linda population.

So, to return to the car analogy, it seems careful driving and regular maintenance are everything. Caring for your physical health is important, but so is your spiritual health. The two go hand in hand.

It's all connected

The idea that our physical health and our spiritual well-being go hand in hand might seem novel in the context of Western medicine, but as you can see from the Blue Zoners it's hardly new. Many of us have long known that health is about more than just the body.

Here in New Zealand, we have our own example in the traditional Māori view of health. One way the Māori 'whole being' view of health is illustrated is through te whare tapa whā, in which the wharenui – with its strong foundations and four equal sides – symbolises the four dimensions of Māori well-being: taha tinana (physical health), taha wairua (spiritual health), taha whānau (family health) and taha hinengaro (mental health). In this model, health and well-being are not measured individually. Community is important, as is having a strong sense of who you are, where you fit in and where you've come from. There is huge sense and merit to this holistic model, and its benefits are borne out in practice. Māori have been found to age positively when they are socially connected and able to serve others. When they have a sense of purpose and are held in esteem and included.

Geriatrician Hamish Jamieson says many people gain from having some sort of spiritual connection. We *all* need to learn to value our ancestors, he says, value where we are and where we've come from. Gratitude and appreciation for our roots is grounding and calming. We thrive, he says, when we are connected.

Connecting with the spirit is something Western society in general has lost. There is lots more to good health than food and exercise. And this tendency in Western medicine to want to force the physical and the spiritual apart has had dire consequences for many cultures. Here in New Zealand, for many Māori, our current health services fail to account for taha wairua, and that's evident in the health outcomes.

I've said that one 65-year-old is vastly different from another, that 'old people' are not one homogenous group. We are also not a classless group. There's a complex collection of circumstances that go into determining how well we age, and things like sexism, racism, poverty, disability and stress all have a part to play. Here in New Zealand, our history of colonialism continues to cause harm. If you are Māori, your life expectancy is seven years less than the average life expectancy. Māori have higher rates of dependency and disability. Most (if not all) have experienced racism in some form – present in even the smallest interactions, such as the doctor who doesn't pronounce your name correctly. It doesn't take a moment to check pronunciation, to make an attempt. It's a matter of care and respect.

The healthcare system, like so many other parts of society, has overlooked Māori needs for too long. We know that Māori do best in the health system when a holistic approach, considering medical, psychological, social and spiritual matters, is used. And, it would seem, everyone else would do better with such an approach, too. In particular, Māori flourish in healthcare when they are able to have whānau around them for support. This also happens to be true for Pasifika people. 'You will rarely see a Pasifika patient alone,' Otago University geriatrician Xaviour Walker tells me. 'Family will be there, sleeping outside ICU on a mat, or even under the bed if need be. It's a matter of honour. It is seen as a shame on your family if you haven't been able to care for your elders.'

Language can pose a huge barrier to access, alienating Pasifika people further from the health system. 'A lot of people are not confident in public settings. Many older people have poor English, they will just sit there and not speak,' Fijian doctor Iris Wainiqolo says. 'People are shy, trying to understand. They will take relatives with them if they need to go to the chemist, or the doctor. There's safety in numbers.'

So, although the research shows it's important to take a holistic view of health and well-being, actually putting those values into practice in our lives can be challenging. It's not entirely up to each of us as individuals; society needs to do its bit, too. After all, it's not a level playing field. It's not our 'fault' if we reach retirement in a physically, mentally or economically vulnerable position.

Our health and well-being is not just our personal responsibility. It is also the responsibility of our community. Other cultures already know this. The Western world would do well to take note.

The bright side

When Jeanne Calment died in August 1997, she was exactly 122 years and 164 days old. According to official records, she remains the only person verified to have lived beyond the age of 120.

Born in Arles, France, before the invention of the light bulb, Jeanne outlived her husband, her daughter and her grandson. At the age of 85, she took up fencing, and was still cycling at 100. She lived on her own until 110, only moving to a nursing home after a fall in which she broke her leg.

Jeanne woke at 6.45 every morning to say her prayers, thanking God for being alive and for the beautiful day. She would listen to the radio, then spend her afternoons visiting others in the home to tell them the news she'd heard. Her diet was rich in olive oil and she loved spicy and fried food. Every day, she enjoyed a fruit salad of banana and orange – as well as an after-dinner glass of port and a cigarette. Her philosophy on life: 'If you can't do anything about it, don't worry about it.'

When it comes to keeping happy and well, it turns out our mind is our most powerful tool. If you are optimistic and grateful, your body will reflect those thoughts. If Jeanne Calment's not proof of that, I'm not sure who is!

Renowned gerontologist Dame Peggy Koopman-Boyden tells me it's a fact: glass-half-full people do live longer, despite the health issues they may have. Specifically, optimists have been found to live longer, have fewer heart issues and not suffer as much depression. In fact, one Harvard study of almost 160,000 women aged between 50 and 79 suggested optimistic women will live more than five per cent longer than their less-optimistic counterparts and are more likely to live into their nineties. What's not to love?

We'll look at this in more depth in Part 2 of this book, but for now all you need to remember is that it's about simple stuff.

- Instead of saying, 'What a ghastly day it is!' Koopman-Boyden suggests trying, 'I love these stormy days! What a great opportunity to stay inside with a good book.'
- Smile at people! They will generally smile back. A smile costs nothing, and can achieve so much.
- Try to think of silver linings.
- Keep a gratitude journal – focus on all the things that are *not* wrong with your life.
- Be kind to others.
- Surround yourself with people who lift your spirits.
- Learn to accept the things you can't change – just like Jeanne Calment.

I know, it all sounds very Pollyanna-ish! However, as I have often told my children and grandchildren, it's OK to fake it till you make it. The brain is a particularly malleable organ. The more you practise optimism, the more your brain will see the world that way.

It's worth it in more ways than one. As well as improving your general sense of well-being, a rosy outlook will help you to eat well and exercise well. In other words, let your mindset lead the way, and your body will follow.

2

THOUGHT FOR FOOD
Eating well

'Let food be thy medicine and medicine be thy food.'
—Hippocrates

Our biological evolution might have taken place very slowly, over the course of many hundreds of thousands of years, but the society and technology we enjoy today have evolved at lightning speed. And one of the major ways the modern Western world differs from times gone by is in terms of our diet.

While our hunter-gatherer predecessors had to work hard for their food, these days we have easy access to pretty much anything our stomachs desire. We can practically inhale thousands of calories in one sitting. Fatty food no longer requires miles of hunting and scavenging, just a short trip to the kitchen or the local fast-food outlet. According to Wayne State University psychiatry professor Arash Javanbakht, 'It is like giving full fridge privileges to your Labrador.' Easy calories, he explained in a 2019 piece for *The Conversation*, give large amounts of energy in a short time, but confuse our whole digestive system.

As a species, we evolved to be active. We often walked many kilometres every day, as well as chasing prey, fleeing predators and shifting rocks. We were not built to sit at a desk or lie on the couch for hours on end, snacking on high-calorie food that came in a bag. It might be tempting to eat whatever we want, whenever we want, but as the old adage goes, 'you are what you eat'. Good nutrition plays an important role at all stages of life, and this is especially true as we age, because our metabolism begins to slow. Your metabolism is the way your body burns calories, converting the food and nutrients you consume into the energy you need to function. How fast your metabolism works is determined mainly by your genes, but you can help it along with a healthy diet and exercise.

Age is not a time of inevitable mental and physical decline, and the food you eat will do much to fuel a healthy lifestyle. It's also not just about what you eat, but how you eat.

Food for thought

Let's start with the how. The good news is, there's nothing especially complicated about it. So long as you follow the old rule of 'everything in moderation', you'll be on the right track! Gary Fraser, the director of one of the aforementioned Loma Linda Adventist Health Studies, has some salient words of advice, gleaned from those years of study.

- **Make dinner your smallest meal.** Have a sizeable breakfast, a good lunch and a smaller evening meal.
- **Fast overnight.** An overnight stretch of 12 to 14 hours free of food will help you keep that 'older-age spread' off.
- **Eat after exercise** rather than before.
- **Focus on your food.** Avoid reading or watching television while eating. It's so easy to slip into that 'dinner on your knees in front of the news' thing, but it turns out your eyes are reflexively linked to digestion. Focusing on your food will help digestion. Really look at your food; zero in on its taste, texture and smell. This will stimulate the release of your digestive juices and encourage your gut to work better.

It's also of paramount importance that you ensure you eat enough. Sadly, malnutrition is common in older age, and with weight loss comes light-headedness and muscle weakness, both of which can increase the risk of falls.

Try not to skip meals, and make sure you eat enough protein – many older people don't. Both protein and fat are important in older age. As we hit our sixties, we need to have a bit of meat on our bones, and we need to hold on to that meat! As University of Auckland professor Ngaire Kerse will tell you, it's important to spread your intake of protein across the day. Eggs are perfect, she says, as are baked beans. (Music to my husband Chris's ears – he can't get enough of them!) Planning regular healthy snacks will also help maintain your weight.

The research shows that, if you're able to eat with someone else, you will eat more. I know this isn't always possible. It can be hard to summon the enthusiasm to rustle up a meal if you're on your own. Whenever Chris is away and I'm home alone, I tend to opt for the easy fix – avocado on toast or an omelette. That's where a meal-box subscription can come in handy. It'll provide the ingredients and the ideas, so you don't have to worry about thinking of something to make. What's more, you might learn how to cook something new. It could even be fun! It's worth checking out the different providers, as they are often competitively priced and can actually be surprisingly affordable.

One of the best ways I know to show love is by cooking a great meal. I am by no means a spectacular cook, but when it goes well, and family and friends gather around a table and appreciate it, there's nothing finer! Summer heralds the arrival of the long 'Italian' lunch at our house. We decorate a table outside with flowers and greenery from the garden, we ponder the menu – not elaborate but yummy, generally a chilled soup like gazpacho, a chicken dish, a simple salad, some fresh baked bread and red wine, with a decadent pud to follow (not the best for the blood pressure, but hey … on the odd occasion!) – and we take our time. Heaven! In the winter, we light the fire, slow-cook a casserole, find the candles, and similar magic happens.

There really is something special about gathering around a table with people you love, and not rushing.

Healthy eating

When it comes to what to eat, the so-called Mediterranean diet – inspired by the eating habits of those who live near the

Mediterranean Sea – is widely held to be a healthy choice. According to the American Heart Association, it may reduce the risk of cardiovascular disease and type 2 diabetes.

As an overview, it's high in:

- olive oil
- legumes (such as beans, peas, lentils and chickpeas)
- unrefined cereals (such as wholegrain or multigrain bread, brown rice, quinoa and oats)
- fruits and vegetables
- nuts.

It also features moderate to high levels of fish and a moderate amount of dairy, and is low in red meat.

So, what else should you eat?

- **Highly coloured foods**. They tend to be beneficial – think blueberries, turmeric and capsicums.
- **Factor in fibre.** Found in wholegrain wheat, wheat bran, rice bran, vegetables, nuts and seeds, fibre draws water into the stools, making them easier to pass – a key factor in maintaining a healthy bowel. Health organisations worldwide recommend 25 to 40 grams of fibre per day. To put that in perspective, one apple contains around 2.4 grams of fibre, there are 8 grams in a bowl of porridge, and a cup of good old multipurpose lentils contains 16 grams!

- **Include foods high in omega-6 and omega-3 essential fatty acids.** The body doesn't make these, so we need to find them in our diet. Omega-3 is found in walnuts, linseeds, soybean oil, canola oil, dark-green vegetables and oily fish. Omega-6 is found in eggs, fish, poultry and soybeans.
- **Hydrate with H$_2$O.** Four to five glasses a day flush the kidneys, ensuring waste and toxins are eliminated from the body. As a rule of thumb, allow about 1 litre of water per 25 kilos of body weight – for instance, if you're 85 kilograms, that's 3.4 litres. If you're not used to drinking that much, make sure you build up to the right amount gradually. Otherwise, you'll always be running to the loo!

Seek out the following:

- **Broccoli.** It's an excellent detoxifier and contains powerful antioxidants.
- **Kale.** Often referred to as one of the world's healthiest foods! It contains lutein, which helps protect the eyes from macular degeneration. It's also an anti-inflammatory food (see 'Good Gut' on page 34).
- **Spinach.** Packed with vitamins, including A, B6 and C, spinach also contains magnesium, calcium and iron. And yes, it does build muscle strength! Remember Popeye? It turns out spinach contains a compound called coenzyme Q10, which aids in muscle strengthening.

- **Nuts.** These provide high levels of protein and are chock full of vitamins and minerals, such as vitamin A and zinc.
- **Beans and pulses.** A great source of fibre, they also help reduce 'bad' cholesterol. Edamame (soybeans) and black beans, in particular, are full of magnesium.
- **Berries.** As well as containing vitamin C and antioxidants, berries are full of prebiotics that promote a healthy gut (see 'Good Gut' on page 34).
- **Avocados.** These store high levels of healthy fats that promote energy, and are also great sources of vitamins C, B6 and folate.
- **Garlic.** It will give your immune system a boost and may help reduce blood pressure.
- **Salmon.** Rich in omega-3 fatty acids (good fats!), it's also high in B vitamins and a great source of protein.
- **Lemons.** One lemon contains about half your daily requirement of vitamin C (which, among other things, helps promote collagen growth in the skin).
- **Kūmara.** Another great source of fibre, kūmara also promotes gut health and supports vision.
- **Red capsicums.** They're full of antioxidants and boost white blood cell growth.
- **Watercress.** Rich in vitamin C and beta-carotene, this is another powerful antioxidant.
- **Cumin.** It's anti-inflammatory and fights bacteria and parasites.
- **Chia seeds.** Add them to your cereal in the morning. They're rich in minerals and omega-3.

Good gut

It's well established that your overall health is closely tied to the health of your gut. A healthy gut is the key to a healthy you.

The gut is literally your colon or large intestine, and it is a key part of your overall digestive system. Its role is to absorb water and break down waste.

Multiple microorganisms live in the gut. Some of these bacteria are beneficial; others are not. The trick is to get the good bacteria operating at peak efficiency. Fibre is especially important to get the gut functioning well. While antibiotics can be a godsend, it's best to avoid unnecessary courses of them, because they don't discriminate between good and bad bacteria. They just clean both out. That's why chemists will often suggest a course of probiotics to follow your antibiotics.

Healing your gut is not a quick fix. It can take up to six months of healthy eating and drinking to balance out your microbiome (the gut flora or bacteria).

Science shows up to 90 per cent of the body's serotonin is made in the gut. Serotonin, sometimes dubbed the 'feel-good hormone', carries messages between nerve cells in the brain and throughout your body. It plays a part in a raft of body functions, from memory and happiness to body temperature, sleep and hunger. Altered levels of serotonin are linked to irritable bowel syndrome and cardiovascular disease, as well as osteoporosis.

Meanwhile, inflammation in the gut has been linked to depression, anxiety and other mood disorders. Classic signs of inflammation include abdominal pain, chest pain, fatigue, joint pain, sores in the mouth and skin rashes. In this instance, food is indeed thy medicine. You can munch on the following standard healthy go-tos to help reduce inflammation:

- **Leafy green vegetables and fruits.** There's good reason for that 5+ a day campaign!
- **Nuts.**
- **Wholegrains.** Think wholegrain bread, brown rice and quinoa.
- **Fish.** Replace red meat with fish, particularly oily ones like salmon and sardines.
- **Spice up your life!** Spices like turmeric, cayenne and ginger help reduce inflammation. So does garlic. What did we ever do without these flavours?
- **Blueberries, beetroot and capsicum.** All are especially high in anti-inflammatory properties.

Cut out the foods that cause inflammation: cheap fats (think greasy takeaways, pizza and biscuits), highly processed foods, preservatives, chemicals and whey. Generally speaking, if you can't pronounce the ingredients listed, it's best to steer clear of them! Beer and spirits can also increase inflammation, but a glass of red wine (which is full of antioxidants) may help. Avoid lots of cheese (although feta is OK) and steer clear of processed meats such as salami, bacon and ham. Above all, keep the salt in check, as too much sodium is a killer – for flavour, try using lemon or herbs and spices instead. A high salt intake can also lead to high blood pressure, heart disease and stroke. (My GP has it top of his list of things to avoid!)

I confess I've been addicted to salt, happily slathering my food with it. I've recently cut my intake right down. It's amazing how quickly your taste buds adjust.

Many health researchers recommend limiting caffeine. As a devotee of a triple-shot flat white, this doesn't sit well with me! I know they're right, but I do love my coffee. The best thing to do is limit the amount you have. In other words, keep it to one really good brew a day. And don't think you can replace the coffee you've forsaken with tea, as it also contains caffeine. Those of us with British heritage will all be familiar with the 'when in doubt, have a cup of tea' frame of mind. Try herbals. And of course, don't forget the water! Keeping well hydrated is great for pretty much everything.

Finally, if you want to keep it really simple, just beware the four white devils:

- white sugar
- white flour
- processed dairy (such as ice cream, flavoured milk or sweetened yoghurt – basically, dairy that has had sugar or other things added)
- table salt.

A word on plant-based diets

According to Gary Fraser, the Adventist Health Studies have provided a marvellous opportunity to study the difference between vegetarians and non-vegetarians. The Loma Linda Adventists all lead similar lifestyles, but half of them are vegetarian. When the studies began in the 1950s, a plant-based diet was not favoured by those in the medical profession. There were concerns around a lack of iron in the diet. Those concerns have since been widely dismissed.

Cancer, dementia and other age-related diseases can be caused by inflammation, and plant-based diets are anti-inflammatory. As Fraser explained to me, blood tests of the Loma Linda vegans (who take things a step further than most vegetarians, consuming no animal products whatsoever) versus non-vegetarians found significant differences in C-reactive protein – a marker of inflammation. The vegans had lower values than non-vegetarians. Furthermore, non-vegetarians had chemicals in their bloodstream (which were literally bathing their cells) that were in quite different concentrations to the vegans, and often this seemed to be reflected in their health outcomes. For instance, the vegans had a 25 per cent lower risk of breast cancer and prostate cancer than the non-vegetarians, and all vegetarians had 15 to 20 per cent less colorectal cancer than non-vegetarians.

Vegetarian diets are often high in nuts, and studies have found nuts are extremely protective against cardiovascular disease. The Loma Linda vegetarians studied, for instance, ate about a handful of nuts four to five times a week, particularly walnuts, almonds and pistachios.

They also avoided processed food. Researchers have found there is a 25 per cent increase in mortality if you eat highly processed food – and, as Fraser wisely notes, plant-based meat alternatives are also highly processed. Processed meat is also very high in sodium.

Supplements

I have, like many people, spent a truckload of cash on vitamins over the years. Most of them I take religiously for a few weeks … before my enthusiasm trails off and there they sit, forgotten and taking up cupboard space till well past their use-by date, until eventually I toss them out. What a waste! Personally, however, I remain a big fan of herbal remedies and believe they provide lots of benefits.

That said, the general advice is that a healthy diet and plenty of fresh air and exercise will do you more good than a bootload of supplements. However, after the age of 50, it turns out the body needs more vitamins and minerals than it did before. So a little boost may well help. There are two vitamins that Fraser recommends.

The first is vitamin B12, the absorption of which is not as efficient as we age. We need B12 to produce red blood cells. They're the ones that carry oxygen to our organs. A deficiency of B12 can make you feel exhausted, and it can also cause pins and needles, dizziness and anxiety. It's also implicated in vision and memory problems. A lack of B12, Fraser says, can even aggravate a tendency towards dementia. So B12 is a big one.

The second is vitamin D. As we get older, the skin is less able to soak up D-rays from the sun, leading to osteoporosis and brittle bones.

There are also other supplements you might find helpful. For instance, I take magnesium. As well as being particularly helpful to encourage a good night's sleep, I find it's also great for muscle cramps and restless leg syndrome. What's more, it has the added benefit of being good for cardiovascular health and reducing inflammation.

Remember the basics

Keep it simple!

- Steer clear of additives.
- Keep it fresh and colourful.
- Avoid the four white devils.
- Eat moderately – generally, portions should fit in the palm of your hand.
- Eat slowly.
- Don't skip meals.
- And try to eat your evening meal early, between 5 and 6 pm, then fast through till breakfast to give your blood sugar time to rebalance during the night.

3

IN OUR CUPS
Drinking

*'There's more refreshment and stimulation in a nap,
even of the briefest, than all the alcohol ever distilled.'*
—Ovid

It's been a bit of a ritual in our house, that quiet drink at the end of the day. My dad loved his gin at lunchtime, and a scotch or two in the evening, followed by a McWilliams Bakano with dinner (it was a rough old red ... New Zealand's wine industry's come a long way since the 1960s!).

I guess I've followed suit. It began with a glass or two of wine to get through zoo hour with the kids, or a good stiff gin while we watched the news. A wee drop of scotch to warm us, a tot to calm the nerves or settle us after a tough day at the office or before a big performance. But how quickly and how insidiously those one or two drinks can become three or four or more.

Lotta Dann became a household name when she confessed, on national television, that she had a drinking problem. Her story on TVNZ's *Sunday* programme struck a chord with thousands of women around the country. There she was – a successful journalist, mother of three boys, married to TVNZ's then-political editor Corin Dann – admitting she was an alcoholic. Lotta says she hears that a lot – the idea that you can appear to have it all together, but underneath you know you're miserable. 'I have a litany of stories of being drunk and falling over and making a fool of myself, but still holding it together and having a life,' she says.

It took an enormous amount of courage to go public, and Lotta did us all a great service. She started an honest conversation about how we are drinking, and the national picture isn't pretty.

The boozey truth

Here in New Zealand, so many of us drink alcohol – and do so regularly – that it seems normal, but is it?

As the NZ Drug Foundation's 2022 *State of the Nation* report stated, 'A large proportion of New Zealanders drink alcohol in a way that causes them harm.' Overall, of the adults surveyed who reported drinking, 25.4 per cent had done so hazardously in 2020–21 – that means over 800,000 of us displayed a regular pattern of drinking with a high risk of future damage to our physical or mental health. While this sort of drinking behaviour was less pronounced in those over 65, it was still of concern.

Alcohol Healthwatch reports that New Zealanders spend upwards of $85 million a week on booze. One joint study conducted by Auckland and Massey universities found Kiwis over 50 are drinking more heavily than their contemporaries in other countries. We're drinking, it seems, on a par with older Britons, but four times more often than the average American. Many assume excessive drinking is a problem of youth, but in fact the latest figures from Figure.NZ show nearly 20 per cent of older men are drinking hazardously. According to the latest figures at the time of writing, New Zealanders 45 and older make up 41 per cent of hazardous drinkers. Worryingly, there has also been a significant increase in out-of-control drinking among older New Zealanders. For those aged 65 to 74, it almost doubled in the four years between 2012 and 2016. You'd think we were old enough and wise enough to know better.

Safe drinking

The precise amount of alcohol a person can drink before it's deemed hazardous varies. As the Ministry of Health/Manatū Hauora bluntly states, 'There is no amount of alcohol that is considered safe and drinking any alcohol can be potentially harmful.'

In order to determine whether drinking is hazardous or not, the NZ Drug Foundation uses a ten-question Alcohol Use Disorders Identification test, which looks at the amount of alcohol a person consumes as well as adverse consequences related to drinking and dependence on alcohol. A person's drinking is considered hazardous if they receive a score of eight or higher.

Generally speaking, less is always more when it comes to alcohol. As the Drug Foundation explains, each person's tolerance for alcohol is different and it's important to know your own limits. It's also important to ensure you eat well and stay hydrated if you're going to be drinking – alternating your alcoholic drinks with glasses of water is a great rule of thumb! The Ministry of Health advises limiting the amount of alcohol you drink, noting that everyone should have at least two alcohol-free days a week, and it's better if those days are consecutive to give your liver more time to recover. When we do drink, the advice is for women to consume no more than two standard drinks a day and men no more than three.

It's also worth remembering that alcohol can interfere with medications you may be taking, either making them less effective or causing them to act far too well. Paracetamol, anti-inflammatories, antidepressants, antibiotics and heart medications are all affected by alcohol. What's more, people of European descent produce more of the enzyme that metabolises alcohol than people of other ethnicities, so if you're not of European descent you may feel the effects of alcohol more than someone who is.

So what is a standard drink? The Ministry of Health guidelines say for spirits it's 30 millilitres – that's about a finger and a half's width of straight spirits. For wine it's 100 millilitres – in a standard stemmed glass, that's filling the glass to its widest point (about halfway). And for beer, it's 330 millilitres, or one tall glass. The standard drink equates to what the average person can process in an hour.

Alcohol and ageing

As we age, exercising restraint when we drink is certainly in our best interests, as alcohol abuse consistently predicts poor ageing.

One of the key reasons for this is that alcoholism damages social supports. It also affects just about every system in the body, its tiny invasive molecules travelling happily all over the place. Older people are particularly at risk of its ravages. As we age, the organs that metabolise alcohol begin to shrink, so alcohol stays in the system for longer. Also, the total fluid in our bodies declines. In other words, we get dehydrated more easily as we age, so the alcohol is more concentrated and won't break down as rapidly as it did when we were 20. That explains why we feel so dusty after a night on the turps. Furthermore, with dehydrated skin comes flakiness and puffy eyes. Not pretty.

Alcohol is a depressant, working its way through the blood–brain barrier. According to Paul Wallace, emeritus professor of primary healthcare at University College London, alcohol has a depressing effect on judgement, planning and reasoning. It may lead to a carefree feeling, but he warns that feeling is short-lived! Something that felt like a great idea when you were chatting over a few wines might not seem so great the next morning. Prolonged drinking, Wallace says, makes you more likely to have mood problems like anxiety and depression.

Alcohol.org.nz notes that alcohol also has the potential to ravage the skin. Over time it can lead to enlargement of the blood vessels and cause unseemly thread veins on the skin's surface, particularly on the face. It also produces a stress reaction that results in an excess of androgen hormones, which aggravates acne.

Beer and wine both contain sugar, and when we consume them in high quantities this can actually damage our skin's collagen and DNA, which of course leads to premature ageing. And, on top of all that, research shows women who drink have a higher risk of developing rosacea.

There are multiple detrimental health effects associated with drinking too much. Binge drinkers – those who consume double the daily limits noted previously – dramatically increase their risk of stroke and heart attack, as alcohol raises blood pressure. It can also damage the heart's ability to pump, increasing the risk of heart failure. Heavy alcohol consumption over a long period of time can also lead to cirrhosis, or scarring of the liver, which prevents the liver from working properly. And in men, excessive drinking can lower testosterone levels and reduce sperm quality and quantity.

Ever wondered where beer belly comes from? The sugar in alcohol raises insulin levels, and turns on fat storage. In middle age, that can result in fat being stored around the tummy. Alcohol also supresses the hormone leptin, which controls the appetite, so it's easy to overeat while drinking.

Our livers aren't the only organs at risk – the brain can actually be affected by alcohol much earlier. Before doctors see liver damage, people might display other symptoms like poor impulse control, anger issues, moodiness or depression, and difficulty making complex decisions, for instance around financial matters.

In terms of cancer risk, it is safest not to consume any alcohol at all. While some studies have shown that moderate drinking – for instance, a glass of wine with dinner – may be beneficial and protect against dementia, there is still debate over those findings. And it now appears that those study results may have been skewed by the participants' wealth and habits that aided good health, such as exercise.

Each year in the UK, there are 13,000 cases of cancer attributed to alcohol. The types most commonly linked to alcohol are mouth, oesophagus, bowel, breast and throat cancer. It's the ethanol that does it – it's broken down by the body into acetaldehyde, which damages DNA and affects the cells that cause cancer.

There is some good news here: if you are already a heavy drinker, all is not lost. It's possible to reverse some of the damage by stopping drinking. The liver, for instance, has the capacity to repair itself, and has been shown to do so after as little as six months off the booze. And, even if you only enjoy the occasional tipple, it's worth knowing that the British Liver Trust recommends three consecutive alcohol-free nights a week to give the liver a chance to repair and regenerate – note this is one more night than the Ministry of Health recommends.

Water: The elixir of life

Fortunately, there's one refreshing and nourishing drink we can enjoy as often as we want: water!

Our bodies are mostly water – around two thirds of the adult human is H_2O. Every cell, every piece of tissue, every organ needs water to function properly. For instance, being well hydrated helps the heart to pump blood around the body. Your heart beats on average 72 times per minute. However, if you're short on water, the amount of blood circulating round the body will decrease, and the heart will have to beat faster to compensate, placing stress on that vital organ.

As we get older, however, our sense of thirst diminishes. This is partly why it becomes much easier to get dehydrated. What's more, as we age, the water levels in the body decrease. So that refreshing tall glass of water has never been more important!

Dehydration can be particularly dangerous for older people, and can mimic the warning signs of dementia. Three quarters of the brain is water. Prolonged dehydration causes the brain cells to shrink, affecting memory and cognition. So, a lack of water can cause confusion, headaches, fatigue and dizziness. This is increasingly common with older people, many of whom have been dehydrated for years through not drinking enough water.

Your joints need water to lubricate them, which is another reason mobility issues become more common as we age. Additionally, older people who are short on water can be prone to urinary tract infections, as the kidneys don't function as well. Dehydration can also lead to gastritis and acid reflux, as the pH levels in the stomach rise. All of which are great reasons for making sure you drink plenty of water!

And there's more! Water increases your energy levels, helps with weight loss (because you can burn more fat), flushes out toxins, improves your skin and keeps you from becoming constipated.

There is no simple rule about how much water a person should drink each day. The precise amount depends on a multitude of factors, including body weight, metabolism, diet, climate and so on. However, most experts agree that somewhere around 2.5 litres a day is about right.

If you find water a bit boring on its own, try adding a couple of slices of cucumber, lemon or lime. Try to drink a glass first thing in the morning, as you will probably have lost water during the night – as well as having gone a good few hours without a drink, you also sweat while asleep.

And don't wait until you're thirsty to drink. By that point, you are already dehydrated. The best indicator of healthy hydration is straw-coloured urine. If the urine is dark yellow, it's time to drink up!

4

MOVE IT OR LOSE IT
Exercise

'Let us cherish and love old age; for it is full of
pleasure if one knows how to use it.'
—**Lucius Annaeus Seneca, *Letters from a Stoic***

Nancy Meherne was a legend around Christchurch's beachside community of Sumner. At the age of 92, she was still a keen bodysurfer, and would cycle the three blocks from her house to the beach to check out the waves.

'I like to see a nice big one coming and a gap,' she told the *Guardian* at the end of 2021. 'You can't get on one little wave after another. You wait until you see a big wave and then you come in on that. I love just speeding in. You're moving so quickly, it's really good.'

Nancy lived for the ocean, and as one of her (much younger) fellow surfers noted, she 'aged but never got old'. As well as being a vegetarian and cutting out sugar, she went to exercise classes and danced to keep supple. Those who knew her talked often of her zest for life and her kindness. When Nancy died at the age of 93, she was surrounded by her family, having lived life on her terms. 'You've got to have fun,' she said.

Meanwhile, in 2022 at the age of 94, Keith Partridge – also from Christchurch – was still running up and down his driveway every day to collect the paper. In addition, he was doing jumping jacks and press-ups twice a day, and cycling about town on an e-bike. He told *Stuff* that keeping active was part of what had allowed him to stay well and living in his own home, even at an age that he himself admitted was 'getting a bit ancient'! Keith never drank alcohol or smoked, and loved his workshop and his garden. Needless to say, he was a favourite with his 14 grandchildren and great-grandchildren!

Both Nancy and Keith are examples of older people who are out living. And, in the process, they're also outliving many of their contemporaries! They are out there enjoying life, keeping active, staying fit.

Another case in point is the many cycling clubs popping up all over the country for people in their sixties and beyond – there's the Rusty Rims, the Grey Spokes, the Whispering Wheels and the Latte Ladies, to name but a few. The Rims riders are mostly in their mid- to late-seventies, and at the time of writing the Whispering Wheels boasts one member who's 91!

We need to be actively encouraging all 50- to 70-year-olds to get fit. As the saying goes, 'work out today, wake up tomorrow'.

Similarly, as Canadian writer and leadership expert Robin Sharma said, 'If you don't make time for exercise, you'll probably have to make time for illness.'

Regular physical activity should be part of everyone's life, and this is especially true as we age. It is good to raise a sweat and get the heart rate up. What's more, as you get older, maintaining a healthy weight remains as important as ever.

Listen to your body!

Many people don't understand how ageing impacts their body, says Hamish Jamieson, an associate professor at Otago University's Christchurch campus and specialist in older persons' health. Jamieson has led multiple studies into better ageing, and he says that as we age, there are whole-body changes to be aware of.

Most of our organs are at peak efficiency in our twenties and thirties, and from there on there is a progressive loss of efficiency over time. This is completely normal. The medical term for it is sarcopenia, and it results in an array of charming physical 'adjustments'!

- The muscles don't work as well, so exercise becomes harder to do, and your pace of walking slows.
- The liver and kidneys also become less efficient, so detoxing takes longer.
- You become tired more easily.
- The heart doesn't beat as fast.

As I said, this is all completely normal. Of course, everyone ages differently – it depends on other factors, such as whether you have an illness, chronic disease or disability, or more generally how much you abused your body in your youth!

While exercise is good and will slow the ageing process, Jamieson warns that you shouldn't be too hard on yourself, even if you think you're pretty fit. In other words, don't expect your 70-year-old body to do what your 30-year-old body did! Exercising, Jamieson says, is great for reducing falls and fractures, and it improves mood and balance, but it's not one size fits all. He recommends getting some advice about your exercise regime from your doctor, particularly if you're planning on resistance training. I know it's tempting in a class to try to keep up with the young ones, but it's much better – and ultimately more effective – if you just listen to your body and work at your own rate.

The good news is there are many programmes out there that are designed to keep older people active, and they can be an excuse to kill two birds with one stone: you get out and get active at the same time as socialising and having fun! As you'll read later, nurturing relationships is a critical component of health and well-being as you age, so any opportunity to do just that is a good one.

Mama Keni Moeroa, an energetic Cook Islands health worker, is still playing competitive netball at 60. 'You're as young as you feel,' she tells me, although she notes that she does get some pushback from older Cook Islanders when she asks them to join an exercise group. 'Oh no, we're too old,' they tell her, as if exercise is only for younger people. Keni has found a way around the reluctance. 'Laughter is the best medicine,' she says. 'We come together at the Pacific Trust seniors' group, there's singing and dancing, it encourages you to be happy.' There it is, singing and dancing: an important part of island life, and the perfect fitness combo!

When it comes to picking the right activity, think about what you need. Choose carefully and find the right balance. Running, for instance, often results in orthopaedic problems, especially in the knees. However, the muscles around your knees will begin to waste away if you're not active, so you do need to keep working the knees – just don't overwork them. Poor muscle tone around the knees is a leading contributor to falls.

Christine Stephens, a psychology professor at Massey University and part of the Health and Ageing Research Team (HART), reckons 30 minutes a day is achievable for most people. In her research, she's found many New Zealanders are remarkably sedentary – it seems we love the couch! She also says a lot of people feel betrayed by health messages. 'You never do stay young,' she says. 'The betrayal comes when you stiffen up and you've followed all the rules yet you're still stiff.' So you're pretty much guaranteed to become a bit stiff as you age. Suck it up! She notes that exercise doesn't have to involve going to the gym, and recommends gardening for the upper body – digging and bending will build strength. What's more, it's good for the soul to be out in nature.

Exercise helps when it comes to maintaining a healthy weight, but again it's a balancing act. Being overweight is related to falls and all manner of diseases, but on the other hand those who are underweight have less in reserve.

What's more, as geriatrician Xaviour Walker highlights, the Western lifestyle – with its 'sugary and fatty fast foods that are cheap and readily available on every street corner' – can have especially detrimental effects depending on your genetic predisposition. According to Walker, who specialises in healthy ageing in Pacific Islanders, this lifestyle has taken a toll on the health of Pasifika people in particular. When you come from places that, throughout history, have been lashed by cyclones and tropical storms that wipe out food crops, your forebears have had to endure long periods with scarce food. Their bodies developed to store what little there was. 'We have been adapting to times of less food because of extreme weather effects for a long time,' he says. 'Now, we're living in an age where we have access to high caloric foods. What's more, lots of cancers are associated with obesity. Maintaining a healthy body weight through exercise and nutrition is extremely important.'

So, exercise helps … but it's just one part of a bigger picture.

A balancing act

Why is it that some of us become prone to falls as we age? I know I'm definitely not as confident on top of a ladder or perched on the roof cleaning out the spouting as I used to be. I find myself feeling a bit wobbly and vulnerable.

I'm not the only one. One in seven New Zealanders 65 and over have a fall each year. Ten to 20 per cent of those people will end up in hospital with a fracture. Interestingly, in Britain, one in three adults over 65 experience a fall each year. Is that possibly because, on average, those in the UK are less likely to be physically active than their Kiwi counterparts?

When does simply 'falling over', which we all do from time to time, become that dreaded 'having a fall'? It turns out it has a lot to do with our ears. The inner ear houses the vestibular system, where we perceive balance. The vestibular system sends messages to the brain which enable spatial awareness and allow us to move confidently. With age, the cells in that system begin to die off, affecting our ability to autocorrect ourselves. So it seems my vestibular system ain't what it was!

Medical conditions like Parkinson's disease, multiple sclerosis and Alzheimer's can also alter your balance, as can some medications. If any of these affect you, talk to your doctor about what is achievable for you when it comes to exercise.

Above all else, be aware of your limitations and take precautions. This is especially true if you've always had good balance in the past, as things may have changed. My 74-year-old husband is a case in point: he recently insisted on clambering about on the roof of our two-storey house to fix the windows. We didn't have a harness, but I'm still quite fond of him, so I insisted on tying a sturdy rope round his middle and attaching it to the bedpost. Do not try this at home! As a nursing friend soberly told me, the spinal unit at Middlemore Hospital is full of older men who thought they were bulletproof. If you must go climbing around on the roof, sturdy scaffolding and a harness are a must.

It's not just our balance that can throw us off, though. Falls become more significant when we become frail.

What is frailty? It's actually a medical term that measures vulnerability to acute injury and how quickly you can recover. Frailty is also based on how many conditions a person is dealing with, as well as their walking speed, grip strength, levels of exhaustion, and weight. Around 20 per cent of New Zealanders over 85 are considered 'frail'.

Sarcopenia, the reduction in muscle tissue as a result of ageing, sets in from age 30. Then, as you enter your forties, bone density begins to deplete, especially in women post-menopause because of the loss of oestrogen, which stimulates bone tissue growth.

But the good news is that frailty is not an inevitable part of ageing – it can be reversed. And if you happen to be diagnosed as 'frail', you can look on it as a challenge to be overcome.

There are a few ways we can avoid becoming frail:

- **Eat lots of fruit and veg.** A study from the *American Journal of Clinical Nutrition* found a link between flavonoids – compounds that are found in fruit and vegetables – and lower rates of frailty onset. Apples and berries are particularly high in flavonoids.
- **Get some vitamin D.** Vitamin D helps strengthen the bones. The best source of vitamin D is sunlight – so be sure to get outside for a few minutes every day. In winter, when there is less sunlight, aim to do an outdoor activity in the middle of the day. Some doctors also recommend taking a vitamin D supplement during these months.
- **Strengthen your muscles.** Try resistance training at least twice a week – you can use weights or just your own body. A Swiss ball is also a great investment! There are many exercises you can try on the ball, from sit-ups to prone leg lifts and lots in between, but go easy at the start if you're

not familiar with exercising on a ball, and get the advice
of a trained Pilates instructor before you begin. A simple
exercise you can start with is sitting on the ball and lifting
one foot off the floor – this will immediately engage your
tummy muscles while you try to balance.

You may feel some apprehension about exercising, particularly
after a fall. If you stop exercising because you're worried about
falling again, a vicious cycle can set in: the fear of falling leads to
no exercise, which leads to loss of muscle, which leads to loss of
strength and balance, which leads to an increased risk of falling!
If you're concerned about injuring yourself, a physiotherapist may
be able to help. They'll show you how to keep those muscles strong
while you ease back into an exercise routine.

Everyday exercises

Our physical strength and bone density peaks when we're around
25 to 30, but happily the decline that sets in around 40 can be
slowed through proper nutrition and exercise. So, how best can we
strengthen our bodies and our sense of balance?

Here are a few everyday tricks that will help:

- **E tu, e noho!** Stand up and sit down! If you are able,
  practise sitting down and standing up without pushing off
  with your hands. Concentrate on using your legs – try not
  to lever yourself up with your arms! Tighten your tummy
  muscles and use your core strength.

- **Lift, hold, repeat.** Stand on your right foot, holding your left leg out at 45 degrees. At the same time, lift your right arm and hold it out at 45 degrees, too. Hold for ten seconds, then repeat with the opposite arm and leg. Try to remain as upright as possible and look straight ahead.
- **Balanced brushing.** Stand on one leg while brushing your teeth. This will strengthen your ankles and improve coordination.
- **Lunge.** Another great exercise for improving balance, lunges will strengthen the whole body, particularly the muscles around the knees and ankles. Remember to have your front knee directly above your ankle and your back knee directly below your hip. Sink down with a straight back, looking straight ahead. It doesn't matter if you can't get down very far to start with. Just make sure the posture's right, and you'll get further with practice.

Work these mini exercises into your day – you can do them while you're standing at the bench making dinner, or getting up from the sofa to search for the remote. All this can be very amusing for your other half or anyone else who catches you at it!

But remember, multi-tasking is bad for your balance. It might be tempting to chat on the phone while balancing a tray in one hand and a pile of washing in the other as you head downstairs … but try to do one thing at a time.

Resistance training, where you make your muscles work against something, can improve muscle strength at any age. You can use free weights, weight machines, resistance bands and even your own body weight to work your muscles and get stronger. British researchers who introduced a ten-week resistance-training course at a rest home for frail older people – some of whom were aged 90 – found a 113 per cent increase in participants' muscle strength. In addition, they also noticed a 28 per cent increase in stair-climbing power and a 3 per cent increase in thigh muscle.

It is never too late to train those muscles. You're never too old to exercise.

Pilates posture

Sporty Spice I am not. I've dabbled with all kinds of keep-fit classes in my time. Remember Jazzercise in the 1980s? All those leg-warmers and big hair? I've also tried aerobics (too hectic), yoga (too slow), running (too exhausting and hard on the knees) and cycling (only now struggling to learn how in order to please my cycle-mad other half!).

But Pilates? Now, that's different. For pretty much the last 20 years, I've been a regular. It's the longest I've stuck with any form of exercise. Somehow, it suits me perfectly. It has just the right combination of strength-building and stretching, and I certainly notice my body seizing up if I don't practise it regularly. What's more, it leaves me feeling both energised and calm (rather than totally exhausted).

Pilates aims to foster a strong mind–body connection, and was the brainchild of German physical-fitness specialist Joseph Pilates. In the early twentieth century, he designed a series of strengthening exercises, and initially focused on rehab for soldiers returning from the war and dancers who were experiencing a lot of aches and pains. Pilates' six original principles remain the foundation of the practice today: centre, concentration, control, flow, precision and breathing.

In Pilates, breath and posture are everything. According to Susie Turner, founder and director of Auckland's Suna Pilates Studio, there are four basic principles to remember for great posture.

1. **Armpits to hips.** Imagine pulling your armpits down towards your hips. This will bring your shoulders down and back, and open your chest. So many of us operate with our shoulders hunched up around our necks, especially those of us who spend the day slaving over a computer.
2. **Belly button to spine.** By pulling your belly button towards your spine, you can correct your pelvic posture. Tilt the pelvis up and forwards, towards your navel. This takes tension off the lower back.
3. **Tattoos out!** Imagine you have tattoos on your inner thighs, and turn them to face outwards. This activates the butt and thigh muscles, and keeps your legs tracking well.
4. **Head lift.** Lastly, imagine you have a thread attached to the top of your head. Allow it to gently pull the head up straight.

And there you have it: the principles of posture. Such a fundamental part of Pilates. Good posture is great for your insides, allowing your internal organs space to sit where they belong, and it's also crucial to a general sense of well-being.

Stress, tension and a fear of the unknown are all part of our daily lives. Many of us are operating in this space, and it just leaves us feeling jittery, lethargic and disconnected from our bodies – basically in fight or flight mode. Pilates is great for this, in that it focuses on breathing as well as exercise.

Good breathing achieves a number of things. For starters, each breath activates the core abdominal muscles, strengthening the abs to take pressure off the back. Furthermore, effective breathing helps kickstart your metabolism, and focusing on the breath (and on the posture) keeps you mindful. You're in the moment and not able to think about anything else. You can work the body and rest the mind.

Piston breathing is a great way to start the day, as it is so quick and easy to do.

- Lean forwards and place your hands on your thighs.
- Fill your lungs by breathing in through the nose.
- Exhale fast through the nose – almost as if you've been punched in the tummy.
- Try to aim for a hundred breaths in rapid succession.

You may feel a bit light-headed to begin with, so take it easy! Once you get the hang of it, it's a sure-fire way to wake up the body and get the metabolism going.

Find the joy

Of course, many of us enter our older years unable to be physically active for a range of reasons. Be kind to yourself. Do what you can achieve. For instance, lunges may be out of the question but arm lifts could be OK. The main thing is to get your doctor's advice about what will work for you – and then be prepared to push it a bit.

Think about why you exercise. Who are you doing it for? Yourself, or someone else? Worldwide, we spend hundreds of billions of dollars a year on weight-loss programmes. Instead, what if we simply focused on finding the right form of exercise for ourselves, so that we could firm and tone the bodies that we have? Wouldn't that be so much better for all of us?

Learn to love the body you're in. After all, it's served you well all these years. Many of us have things we'd like to change about our bodies, but trust me: we'll never look better!

Don't exercise because you fear ageing. Exercise because you find joy in it. Find that joy. It may be walking, cycling, going to the gym, tai chi, Pilates, yoga or classes run by the YMCA. The type of exercise you do isn't what's important; working all the body parts is! Try to work to the point where you're breathing rapidly. Give the cardiovascular system a good old workout. On this front, nothing beats a good brisk walk – around 30 minutes a day is ideal. As well as oxygenating your blood and keeping your brain cells healthy, walking activates the lymphatic system, eliminates toxins, fights infection and strengthens immunity. So bear that in mind next time you're slogging around the block! You'll also find walking reduces anxiety – it's tricky to walk briskly and feel anxious at the same time.

Routine is the name of the game. Make exercise a habit. My mum took up yoga back in the 1960s, and many's the day I came home from school to find her standing on her head in the living room. At the time, I thought she was embarrassingly bonkers – but, looking back, I feel lucky to have had her example to spur me on. I may not have latched on to yoga like she did, but she showed me it was possible to try different things, and that's how I eventually found my thing in Pilates. If you enjoy your exercise, you'll find it much easier to set and keep a routine.

However, if you still struggle to stick with it, there is hope for you yet. My daughter Gemma, probably seeing that my own routine left a bit to be desired, recommended a book called *Atomic Habits*, in which the author, James Clear, suggests there are three laws to establishing a good routine:

1. **Make it obvious.** In my case, I set aside regular time in my diary for Pilates classes. I know where I'm going and when.
2. **Make it attractive.** I anticipate how great I will feel once I've exercised, and how I will finally be able to fit into that pair of jeans that are currently too tight!
3. **Make it easy.** I get my exercise gear, mat, drink bottle, concession card and car keys all ready the night before. No last-minute stress!

Clear reckons people who make a specific plan about when and where they will do something are more likely to follow through. 'People often feel they lack motivation,' he says. 'What they really lack is clarity.'

So, the idea is to say out loud, 'I will exercise for 40 minutes from nine o'clock on Monday, Wednesday and Friday mornings.' Then put it in the diary. That's your time.

Researchers in the UK worked with a group of more than 200 people to build better exercise habits over two weeks. The participants were divided into three groups. The first group was told to track whenever they exercised. The second had to read motivational material about exercise – how it is good for your heart health and so on — and were also told to track their exercise. The third group read the same motivational material, but were asked to make a plan for where and when they'd exercise over the following week. In the first and second groups, about 38 per cent exercised at least once a week. By contrast, in the third group, 91 per cent exercised at least once a week. That's a win.

I'm trying to persuade my husband Chris to create a habit: 'I will make Jude a cup of tea and some toast at seven o'clock every morning and take it to her in bed.'

It hasn't worked so far, but I live in hope! (Though I suspect habit-forming is more successful when it comes from yourself, rather than your wife.)

How much?

Generally speaking, experts recommend 30 to 40 minutes of moderately vigorous activity three to four times a week. Most scientists agree that the more we exercise beyond 60 years of age, and the further past 30 minutes a day of exercise we can get, the more the risk of chronic disease drops, and the longer and healthier our lives will be.

To get more specific, it depends on who you ask and what you're doing. Scientists from the Centers for Disease Control and Prevention in the US recommend those who are physically able and over 65 should do around 150 minutes of moderate exercise per week, or half that if it's intense exercise like running or cycling. They also suggest muscle-strengthening exercises twice a week on top of that, including some exercises for balance.

Apparently, it doesn't matter how you break the exercise up during the week. Short bursts more frequently are equally as effective as longer chunks less often. What's more, simple everyday tasks count. Take the stairs not the elevator, do the vacuuming, lift the heavy shopping bags! I recently interviewed Jo Morgan, who is renowned for her motorcycle adventuring, for taking up mountaineering at 58 and for going on to summit more than 20 peaks. She told me that other mountaineers, many of whom were half her age, were amazed by her strength and agility. How did she maintain that level of fitness? Not in a gym, she says. A keen gardener, she was often found up a tree, wielding a chainsaw. That, and housework!

According to Ulf Ekelund, a professor in the Department of Sports Medicine at the Norwegian School of Sports Sciences, speedy walking five times a week for half an hour will lower your risk of heart disease, stroke, type 2 diabetes and many types of cancer. Ekelund says moderate exercise should increase your breathing and heart rate. On a scale of one to ten, with ten being the most vigorous, moderate should be around six. He recommends picking up the pace a bit, but not so much that you're sprinting!

If you've been diligently counting your steps, consider yourself relieved of that duty. You don't have to achieve 10,000 every day. That's a lot of steps! According to the experts, if you're over 60, around 8000 steps a day is just fine.

There is some bad news, alas. Even 150 minutes of exercise a week may not be enough on its own to keep the weight gain that comes with age at bay. Back in 2010, I-Min Lee, a professor of epidemiology at Harvard's School of Public Health, studied around 35,000 women and found that only those who walked or exercised for an hour a day maintained their ideal weight as they aged. They were the only ones who managed to hold off the old-age spread. That might sound like a lot of exercise, but don't despair! Remember, gardening, walking up and down the stairs, even cruising the shops all count as exercise. Keeping mobile is the thing.

And about that inexorable spread around our middles, a US study found fasting overnight from 5 or 6 pm until 9 the following morning can help to maintain a trim figure. This finding echoes those from the Adventist study.

Anyway, fear of ageing or putting on weight shouldn't be your main reason for exercising. Do it because you enjoy it, because it makes you feel good. Do it for you!

After all, you might want to delay the George Burns effect. 'You know you're getting old,' the American comedian famously said, 'when you stoop to tie your shoelaces and wonder what else you could do while you're down there.'

5

THE GREAT OBSESSION
Sleep

'O sleep, O gentle sleep,
Nature's soft nurse.'
—William Shakespeare, *Henry IV*

I have been obsessed with sleep for decades. Sleep or, more accurately, the lack of it.

It began with babies. Those little bundles of joy that became my night-time tormentors. Until the first one came along, I'd taken my eight hours for granted. Slept like a log. Then, suddenly, we were being awoken three or four times a night. Colic, nightmares, wet beds, high temperatures, mumps, chickenpox, growing pains … You name it, they had it. Eventually they became teenagers, and I'd lie awake waiting for them to come home and then I'd worry about being half asleep on the news the following day – thank goodness for the TVNZ make-up artists, who regularly managed to downsize the black rings under my eyes to almost bearable levels. I haven't really slept solidly for a stretch of nights since. It's been a while. That first baby is now 45!

I'm not alone with my insomnia, if my conversations with other women my age are anything to go by. In fact, during the early days of Covid, my book-club mates and I talked of planning a 2 am Zoom call, fed up as we were with suffering in silence while the other sleeper in our beds snored happily alongside. (I've since discovered that many men are not sleeping as soundly as my other half was on those nights.)

Should we just suck up this lack of sleep and accept it as part of the ageing process? No, say the experts. We need our sleep now, just as we did when we were younger. It is, they say, a key part of our natural toolkit for retaining good health. And yet, a good night's sleep is becoming increasingly elusive in this fast-paced world in which we're living.

Nap tactics

We are constantly bombarded with the message that sleep is vital for our good health. We spend a third of our lives asleep, we're reminded. Everything that has life sleeps, even bacteria. Sleep helps regulate every system in our bodies. It is essential for our immune system. It allows our cardiovascular system to rest and restore itself. Our blood pressure drops during sleep, relaxing pressure on the heart and giving it a well-earned break.

The brain, on the other hand, is particularly active during sleep. Its job is to process and consolidate memories, to deal with the detritus of the day and put it into some sort of order. A vast amount of what we remember is dependent on the quality of our sleep. (No wonder my UE results were so average. Rather than spending every last minute cramming, I would have been better off, the scientists say, to study during the day, then sleep the night before an exam. That would have given my brain the time it needed to consolidate and remember what it had learnt.)

So, we get it. We need sleep. But does it have to be an uninterrupted eight hours? Apparently not. As the University of Auckland's Ngaire Kerse will tell you, a whole night's sleep in one stretch is overrated. 'We have to introduce the idea that it's OK to be awake at night,' she says.

It's society that has pushed us to sleep in one block. Our days have become incredibly structured, driven by the pressures and deadlines of modern living – the need to get to work, to school, to after-school activities, to social outings and so on – and our sleep patterns have changed to accommodate all this hectic activity. Sleep has been squished into a smaller window.

What's more, the 'need' to sleep in one chunk has become commercialised. All those sleep programmes, supplements, pills and potions comprise a multibillion-dollar industry that does little besides fuel our anxieties about getting 'enough' sleep while emptying our pockets. 'A lot of people have lots of anxiety about sleep,' Kerse notes, 'but our ancestors never expected to sleep all night. They'd be up every four hours or so to stoke the fire.'

You may also have heard that as we age, our need for sleep decreases. This isn't true – scientists recommend seven to eight hours – but, as you now know, that sleep doesn't have to come in one stretch. Older people will often experience 'split' sleep, where they'll sleep soundly for the first four or five hours of the night, then wake, only to return to sleep later for another two or three hours. It turns out we naturally wake about ten times an hour, although we're not aware of it. It's our body's natural way of maintaining muscle tone.

Our natural sleep cycle occurs in four stages:

1. **Stage one is the transition phase.** We move from wakefulness to sleep. Our breathing starts to slow and, hopefully, our muscles begin to relax.
2. **Stage two is rest.** Our body temperature drops, our breathing slows further, as does our heartbeat, and there is no eye movement.
3. **Stage three is deep sleep.** Our breath becomes slow and steady. This is the restorative phase of sleep, in which cells are repaired and our immune system is fortified.
4. **Stage four is rapid eye movement (REM) sleep.** The brain becomes more active, and the body cools. This is where most dreaming occurs. Our pulse, blood pressure and breathing speed up. This is an important part of sleep for learning and memory.

A full cycle of these four stages takes approximately 90 minutes to complete. REM occurs between an hour and an hour and a half after falling asleep, and a good night's sleep will last for three or four 90-minute cycles.

As newborns, most of us slept for 14 to 17 hours a day. (I'm emphasising the *day* here, because mine seemed to be awake much of the night!) As teens, eight to ten hours was the gold standard, possibly more, as any parent of teens will tell you. The teen's body clock shifts later, too – they want to sleep in till midday and stay up till 2 am and beyond. For those of us in our seventies, our clock is likely to shift earlier – we move to earlier bedtimes and correspondingly earlier wake-ups. We still, though, need those seven to eight hours.

After lunch, many of us experience a dip in our energy – something Europeans have seized on to justify that most glorious of institutions, the afternoon siesta. My granny, in her eighties, was a great believer in the afternoon nap. She'd take to the couch regular as clockwork straight after lunch. Then she'd wake up perky as and thrash me at canasta. If you, too, like to nod off after lunch, just remember to keep it short – 40 minutes max. Any more, and you'll wake up groggy and it'll interfere with the night's sleep patterns.

Light and dark

As we age, our circadian rhythms change. We feel less refreshed after sleep, we're more likely to wake at night, and we're more likely to feel sleepy during the day. The circadian rhythm is the natural biological clock within the body that regulates the sleep–wake cycle. It also affects hormone release, eating habits, digestion and body temperature. Scientists figured all this out by studying the humble fruit fly which, it turns out, has a surprisingly similar genetic make-up to humans!

Every single cell in our body has a circadian clock, and that clock is governed by light. Exposure to bright light is the most important stimulus for our circadian clock. This is not some wacky theory. It's soundly grounded in science. Bright light supresses the sleep hormone melatonin in the brain, and releases cortisol, making us alert and ready to start the day.

Many people will tell you they sleep really badly around full-moon time. I'm one of them. Personally, I think I may be part werewolf – I'm wide awake during the full moon and frequently feel like howling at it, mainly because of sleep deprivation! Sleep expert Dr Rosie Gibson, from the Sleep/Wake Research Centre at Massey University, says there's no clear cause for sleep to be disrupted around the full moon, but increased light could be part of the story. That or possibly geomagnetic variation caused by the moon, which could be linked with sleep cycles and other health issues such as heart rate variations and migraines. The phases of the moon have also been linked with hormonal cycles and mood disorders. Gibson hastens to add that the evidence for all this is mixed. Whatever the cause, one way I've found of coping with my 'moon problem' is to keep an eye on the silver orb's phases and try not to schedule hectic days when the moon is full.

Māori have long recognised the power the moon has over us, most obviously in the maramataka, the lunar calendar. In the maramataka, each moon phase is linked to certain activities; some phases are better for planting, others for harvesting, and some are reserved for important rituals. As Nic Low wrote in *New Zealand Geographic* in 2022, the maramataka came to Aotearoa with the first explorers from the Pacific. 'They imported Polynesian knowledge earned from millennia spent observing the behaviour of living things in relation to the phases of the moon,' adding that this in turn gives the maramataka a 'predictive power: each day of the month specifies certain activities to seek out, or avoid. This day will be good for fishing. That day will be fair for eels. Those days? Don't bother. Rest.' In other words, the maramataka teaches us there is a strong correlation between energy levels and the phases of the moon.

Light at the right time is a good thing for more than just our sleep routine. Apparently 30 minutes of exposure to bright light in the morning is a powerful antidepressant. No matter how desperately you want to hunker down in bed, the healthy option is to get up, get outside and go for a walk. Get that early morning dose of light into the brain. It's really tempting to reach for your sunglasses first thing in the morning, especially if you haven't got around to patching up those bags under the eyes with a dash of make-up, but really you're best to let that lovely light penetrate your retina uninterrupted.

For older people in care or those with mobility issues, getting outside for some light exposure may not be so easy. However, making sure you can sit near a window in the morning will help. That dose of morning light also plays a role in hospitals. Scientists have found that patients get well faster if their bed is by a window with good access to daylight.

A large part of our body clock is wired into our genes. We tend to fall into two categories: the night owls and the morning larks. I did, on the odd occasion, work on the TV3 breakfast news programme, but after nearly 40 years' working at the other end of the day, it was a stretch for my body clock. You can, however, alter your sleep patterns gradually by exposing yourself to bright light early in the day to wake yourself up. If you want to sleep in longer in the morning, try going for a walk in the light later in the day, which delays the onset of sleep. Or you can stay in bed with the curtains drawn for an extra hour. Denying yourself bright light in the morning will also help shift your wake-up later. Eventually, your body clock will adjust. A similar technique works with jetlag. If it's daylight when you arrive at your destination, make sure you head outside as soon as possible to get that bright light on your retina. Then go to bed reasonably early in a darkened room.

Sleep hygiene

Our cave-dwelling ancestors began to wind down their day with the fading light. Physical activity would cease, giving the brain an opportunity to slow in anticipation for sleep. It is natural for us to take time to prepare the brain for slumber.

One of the most proactive things you can do to get a good night's sleep is to maintain a good sleep routine. This is also sometimes referred to as good sleep hygiene, and is simply about ensuring you've done everything you can to make your bedroom environment and daily schedule compatible with a good sleep. There's no one set way to practise good sleep hygiene, and you can tailor the routine to suit your needs, but there are a few common themes.

- **Stay consistent.** Go to bed at the same time each night and plan to wake at the same time each morning, even on the weekends and on holidays.

- **Keep the bedroom peaceful.** Get rid of the TV in the bedroom to create a calm environment and remove stimulating blue light. Also try to avoid TV for at least an hour before bed – the temptation to binge-watch that drama won't help your sleep. Our brains are not wired for going from intense stimulation to instant sleep. We need to wind down. No surprise then that going straight from that six-part thriller to sleep just doesn't work for us.

- **Turn off the other devices, too.** Stop using them at least an hour before bed, and ideally don't have them in the bedroom when you're trying to sleep. It's well documented that blue light emitted from electronic devices like TVs, computers, tablets and smartphones will interfere with the production of melatonin in the brain, and an abundance of melatonin is what you need for sleep. Blue light mimics the blue we see in the sky, and we are evolved to be awake during the day, so you can see why the brain gets a little confused!

- **Cover your clock or your phone if you use it as an alarm.** Staring at the clock all night long will just make you anxious about the amount of sleep you're missing out on.

- **Warm up to cool down.** You may want to try having a hot shower just before bed, or a hot drink. The reasoning behind this? The body cools after a hot shower, which in turn promotes sleep. As the body warms, we wake up.

The factors that contribute to insomnia are well documented. Stress, disease, poor sleep hygiene and that other old hoary chestnut, 'maladaptive thinking'. That's me! The 'I must get eight hours or I will die!' school of thought.

Pretty much all of us will experience insomnia at some stage or another. The good news, according to Jose Loredo, director of the Sleep Medicine Center at the University of California, San Diego, is that most of us are able to deal with it by ourselves. He has made a study of sleep, and he says it's important to let the brain do what it does. 'Step out of the way and eventually you will recover,' he says. 'Be satisfied with what you've got. Don't worry about not sleeping, start to relax and sleep will come eventually.' Ha! Four hours a night would turn me truly feral, but I'm prepared to give him the benefit of the doubt. The thing is, sleep is about confidence – having confidence that you will sleep, eventually.

According to Loredo, sleeping pills are not the answer – they only encourage dependence. Russell Foster, head of Oxford University's Sleep & Circadian Neuroscience Institute, agrees. Sedated sleep, Foster says, is no replacement for biological sleep. What's more, sleeping pills may affect your memory. Granted, there is a place for them, especially after traumatic events or in extreme cases of insomnia. Using them for a couple of weeks can help get you through a tough time and help reset the body clock. But that's very different from taking them every night for years and becoming completely reliant on them. As well as being highly addictive, they often leave you feeling groggy and disoriented in the morning. They also affect the depth of your sleep, meaning it's not as effective or satisfying. A note of caution here: if you are used to taking sleeping pills regularly, please talk to your doctor before you begin to wean yourself off them. Your doctor will be able to advise the best way to do so safely.

Foster also has a healthy scepticism of sleep apps on smartphones, which usually claim to help you sleep better and wake up feeling refreshed. These apps track and interpret your 'sleep data', and often make outrageous claims – one suggested its users had a 40 per cent deeper sleep, something Foster reckons is biologically impossible. When it comes to the reliability of these apps, Foster recently told *Deep Dive* podcaster Ali Abdaal, 'you'll see [an app] worked perfectly for eight undergraduates in California, and that's about it. But of course … sleep changes as we age and between individuals, and so one algorithm is also not appropriate for telling us what "good sleep" is.'

So, if neither apps nor pills are much help in the long term, what is? Foster advises investing in a good mattress and pillow, and trying to stay calm (for some more tips on that front, see pages 271–275). That way you'll almost always go back to sleep.

It's also important to address the root cause of your sleep problem. What is needed, the experts say, is to understand why you are not sleeping. Is there a genetic predisposition? Is the cause psychological? Or physiological? Are you just 'wired' when you go to bed? And why is it that, when I'm awake at two in the morning, my mind instantly turns to problems?

Rosie Gibson says our brains have a tendency to fall into repetitive negative thought processes rather than positive ones. When we're in bed and less active, we're more likely to notice those thoughts. Also, if we're busy during the day, it may be the only time we have to go over everything that happened in the past 24 hours and collate all our worries. When we're sleep-deprived, our emotional processing is impacted, and we're less able to regulate negative emotions. The answer? Gibson suggests trying to set aside time to address those worries before night rolls around.

About 25 per cent of men have obstructive sleep apnoea, a condition where you stop breathing while you're asleep (some studies show that number is higher, depending on how you define it). Who knew our blokes were suffering so? They sweat, snore and occasionally choke (sound familiar?) and it's a significant public-health problem. And, although sleep apnoea is most common in men, women are also affected, particularly after menopause.

If you're constantly tired and dropping off to sleep during the day, you may well have undiagnosed sleep apnoea. Sleep apnoea sufferers are thought to lose sleep for at least a third of their time in bed. With increasing age, not to mention obesity, airways become floppy, causing them to narrow or even close, and this leads to sleep disruption. Sleep apnoea can be improved with weight loss, aerobic exercise and avoiding alcohol (which relaxes the throat muscles). The most effective treatment for obstructive sleep apnoea appears to be continuous positive airway pressure (CPAP), which is about as sexy as it sounds. A CPAP machine holds your airway open by gently blowing air into your nose and throat, via a mask. And, though it may not be attractive, it is the gold standard and touted as 100 per cent effective.

Snoring can be a deal-breaker in many marriages, so it's worth addressing it early. On the worst nights at our house, I've found it's best to just move to another bed. There's quite a stigma surrounding separate sleeping arrangements for couples, but I know a number who sleep in different bedrooms and it has only enhanced their relationships, so stigma schmigma!

Other tricks

As well as the sleep hygiene practices noted above, there are a few other things you can try in order to promote good sleep:

- **Avoid alcohol for at least two hours before bed.** Alcohol can disrupt the patterns of your sleep. While it may cause you to fall into a deep sleep quickly, you may often find yourself waking again around 2 or 3 am.
- **Beware of diet pills.** These can cause sleeplessness.
- **Keep the bedroom cooler.** Somewhere between 18 and 20 degrees Celsius is optimal. And put the duvet in storage over summer!
- **Put your thoughts elsewhere.** If you find your mind is jam-packed with thoughts (as mine often is), you can try keeping a pen and notebook next to the bed, and writing things down as they occur to you. Alternatively, some people like to visualise putting their thoughts in a box to be dealt with later. The box thing hasn't worked for me, but I do find a notebook incredibly handy. Often my best ideas occur in the middle of the night!

- **Relax.** Breathe deeply in through your nose and out through your mouth, while consciously tensing and relaxing your entire body from the tip of your toes, up your legs, to your torso, arms, hands, neck and head.
- **Try some soothing sounds.** Soft music or white noise, like ocean waves or the sound of rain, can help. There are some great white noise machines out there.
- **Try melatonin supplements.** Melatonin is a hormone that helps with sleep, and your body naturally makes more when it gets dark and stops when it gets light again. It also seems we produce less melatonin as we age. Here in New Zealand, melatonin supplements are only available with a prescription or after consultation with a pharmacist, and it's advised that you only use them for a short time until you re-establish a good sleep habit. Also, make sure you take them at least an hour before bed, otherwise you may feel groggy in the morning.
- **Try magnesium supplements.** Magnesium is vital for overall body function, and can help with both sleep and restless legs. You can usually get enough from your diet, but some people find supplements, which are available in pharmacies and health shops, helpful. Wriggly legs have long been a problem for me – trust me, you don't want to be sitting next to me in a long movie! – but I've found magnesium does help.
- **Ask your doctor about other supplements.** There are some suggestions that tart cherry and iron tablets help with sleep, although the evidence to support this is sparse.

The best thing to do is chat to your GP and see what they think. Personally I have found supplements helpful.

- **Shift your main meal to the middle of the day.** This, at least, was one thing the Covid lockdowns and being stuck at home made easier! Eating a big meal close to bedtime may cause indigestion. If that happens, try my granny's cure: half a teaspoon of baking soda in a small glass of water. Works a treat!

- **Put your wakeful hours to use.** Older Māori often speak of using wakeful times in the night for spiritual reflection and for reconnecting with the past – both with tūpuna and past events. These times can also be a great opportunity to meditate – for more on that, see pages 271–275.

- **Avoid caffeine before bed.** Some people will tell you they can tolerate coffee at night, but research shows that the sleep you get after a cup of coffee is lighter. The same goes for tea and, sadly, chocolate.

- **Get up.** If you wake at around 2 am on the knocker, as I'm prone to do, try this technique from Dr Colin Espie, professor of sleep medicine at the University of Oxford. Just lie quietly with your eyes open. If you're not asleep in 15 minutes, then get up, have a warm calming drink and read a book. Doing so works like a reset, and will almost always help you nod off. This technique seems to work for me!

Sweet dreams!

6

MAINTENANCE
Healthcare

'It is health that is the real wealth,
not pieces of gold and silver.'
—**Mahatma Gandhi**

As we age, there are many things we can do to try to remain as physically healthy as possible. However, even with the best diet, most regular exercise and deepest sleep, bad luck can still strike. Just when you think things are going well, something comes out of left field to blindside you.

When it comes to taking care of your health, you can really only do your best – and then, if the worst happens, try to figure out a way through.

Bad news

Just before Christmas 2018, Chris spotted a tiny pink lump on his forearm. It looked a bit like an insect bite. 'Better get it checked,' I said. The man I married is fair. He burns. He also has a lot of moles on his body.

He duly took himself off to the skin-check clinic. 'Not sure about this one,' his doctor said. 'I think we'll take it off.'

Chris was left with a sizeable scar and about ten external stitches. The excised tissue went off to the lab for testing. Ten days later, he popped into the clinic to get the stitches removed. He rang me from the car afterwards. 'The nurse says it's a melanoma.' My stomach lurched. I could hear the fear in his voice. 'She says the doc will need to talk to me. He'll ring later in the day.' It was a Thursday, and I had work to do, but I couldn't concentrate. Suddenly just one thing, and one thing only, mattered: what would the doc say?

I had to wait a couple of hours before Chris rang me back. 'He wants to see me at five. He wants you to come, too.'

Oh my God, I thought. This is not good.

It turned out that the tiny pink 'insect bite' was in fact a grade-four melanoma. Of the three main types of skin cancer, melanoma is the most serious. It doesn't distinguish between young or old, fit or otherwise. It can spread very quickly, and once it's below the skin's surface (the epidermis), it can rapidly become life-threatening. A grade-four diagnosis meant the doctors were concerned it had spread to other parts of his body – on a scale of one to four, four is the most serious. The doctor confirmed it had already penetrated well below the epidermis, and the question now was whether it had spread to the lymph nodes. And, if so, had it also made it to other organs?

The doctor was extraordinarily patient with our questions, and so kind. 'You know how serious this is?' he said. We did, but we also didn't. 'Do you want me to tell you your chances of survival, Chris?' he asked.

Chris and I looked at each other.

'No,' Chris said. His reasoning: what difference would it make? Even if he was given a 90 per cent chance of survival, he could still be in the ten per cent that didn't make it … or vice versa. Best to just push forward and be as optimistic as possible, he figured.

Our next step was to see a specialist, and we were fortunate enough to get an appointment with Richard Martin, who is widely regarded as the country's leading melanoma surgical oncologist. The only hitch? The appointment wasn't till the following Monday. The intervening weekend was the longest of our lives. Chris and I moved like a couple of zombies on autopilot. We were both very emotional, and could hardly bear to lose sight of each other. All of a sudden, all the plans we had for our future together were on hold. What's more, it was our eldest son's fortieth birthday and he was having a party. We decided to celebrate with him, and keep the news to ourselves until we had more information.

Finally, Monday rolled around and Richard examined Chris's slender forearm. 'I'm going to need to remove a further two centimetres from around this existing wound,' he explained. 'And I'll also need to remove the lymph nodes to check whether the cancer has spread.'

We had to wait a further week for the surgery. In the scheme of things, I know that's not long at all, but it felt like an eternity. We told the kids, and they immediately rallied around to support us. They are all extremely close to their dad, and they were keen to be upbeat and encouraging to help him through. Chris and I tried to carry on as normal, but it was impossible to concentrate. The nights were the worst. Neither of us slept much; instead we just held each other, speaking little, our minds spinning around the worst thoughts in the small hours. We fought the temptation to consult Dr Google. 'Nothing good will come of it,' Richard had told us.

Instead, we tried turning ourselves to more positive things. What could we do that might improve Chris's chances? We began juicing in earnest – beetroot, carrot, celery, ginger, turmeric, garlic and broccoli. We exercised every day. We cut down on red meat and dairy, instead opting for vegetarian dishes with lentils, chickpeas and pulses. We also stopped drinking alcohol – well, mostly. The odd red wine crept in!

Above all, we looked for ways for Chris to reduce stress. His job as the managing director of South Pacific Pictures was demanding – just the sort of thing my husband, who loves a challenge, is naturally drawn to – but it could become all-consuming from time to time. We both knew things needed to change. Chris needed to downsize the job, do fewer hours, take on fewer projects. This was one of the toughest bits of the whole process for Chris to wrestle with. He told me he felt as if he was letting people down by stepping away. I reassured him that the time had come to think of himself and his future.

After the surgery, Chris was left with an impressive scar that runs half the length of his forearm. And Richard had good news for us: the cancer hadn't spread. He was 97 per cent sure that Chris is in the clear. There are no words to describe our relief. It was just monumental. We both felt so very lucky.

While Chris and I remain enormously grateful he dodged that particular bullet, life will never be the same. There's an uncertainty and vulnerability that lingers. What about that three per cent? The man I met and fell for when I was 18, the man I've loved for nearly 50 years, is no longer ten feet tall and bulletproof. He is on three-monthly checks, and at the time of writing is about to have yet another mole removed (there have been numerous 'slices and dices', as we call them, in the intervening years). Needless to say, my heart is in my mouth.

Chris and I learnt a lot from his melanoma scare. We don't take anything for granted. To us, each day is a gift, to be lived to the max. We prioritise the things that really matter: each other, family, friends, health, home. And we would urge you, if you don't already do so, to begin a regular skin-check regime. If possible, go to a mole-mapping clinic or to someone who is able to keep track of any changes to moles you may have. It could save your life.

It helps to know the warning signs. While most moles, brown spots and growths on the skin are harmless, that's not always the case. The ABCDE guide offers a handy way to remember the things to watch out for:

- **Asymmetry.** In most melanomas, the shape of one half is different from the other.

- **Border.** The edges of a melanoma tend to be ragged, notched, blurred or irregular.
- **Colour.** Benign moles are usually just one colour, while melanomas may have different shades of black, brown and tan. And, as it grows, white, grey, red, pink or blue may also appear.
- **Diameter.** Usually, melanomas are at least six millimetres across. (That's about the same diameter as a pencil.)
- **Evolving.** Any change in size, shape or colour or any bleeding, itching or crusting can be a warning sign of melanoma.

Basically, if you notice any variation whatsoever, get it checked. Remember, too, that melanomas can arise on parts of the skin where the sun never shines, such as between your toes and on your scalp. And, above all else, the earlier you get on to it, the better your chances will be.

New Zealand has one of the highest rates of skin cancer in the world, second only to Australia. Around 4000 New Zealanders are diagnosed with melanoma every year, and around 70 per cent of those diagnoses are in people over 50. It's worth taking it seriously.

Be proactive

When it comes to your health, don't just wait for the worst to happen. Take action, and be responsible for getting regular check-ups so you know what's going on. Remember that car analogy? Well, think of this as your health warrant of fitness.

Visit your GP regularly, check your blood pressure and keep up to date with blood tests, smear tests, osteoporosis tests, and so on. In addition, make sure you concentrate on a few key parts.

Ears

Are you always complaining about people mumbling? Do you frequently have to turn up the volume on the TV? Are you always asking people to repeat themselves? At social outings, do you often give vague responses when you haven't heard what's said, nodding and grinning and hoping for the best? I've noticed myself doing all of these things. Which reminds me, I must get a hearing test …

As with all aspects of your health, the sooner you deal with any perceived hearing loss, the better. Most people experience gradual hearing loss as they get older, due to ageing of the inner ear. Loudness and clarity may begin to fade. If this is happening to you, get it seen to. Don't let vanity hold you back. A loss of hearing is one of the leading contributors to the onset of dementia.

In the best-case scenario, you could simply have conductive hearing loss, which can be caused by a build-up of wax in the ear, a perforated eardrum, fluid in your inner ear or even damage to the tiny bones of the inner ear. All of these things can be treated medically or surgically.

On the other hand, it might be that you have sensorineural hearing loss, which is permanent. This is when the hair cells in the inner ear break down so they can't send messages to the brain, resulting in loss of hearing. A hearing aid will help here – and that's better than it sounds! Many modern hearing aids are barely noticeable and make all the difference when it comes to living a socially connected and fulfilling life.

Tinnitus, or ringing in the ears, is very common. Sometimes I feel as though I have an entire colony of cicadas in my ears, the buzzing and humming is so loud. The upside is that it sounds like summer all year round, but it's actually quite tiring – a bit like having the rangehood extractor on all the time. As you get used to it, it becomes an almost subliminal noise, but the silence whenever it does stop is glorious. Tinnitus is sometimes caused by wax and sometimes by a head or neck injury, but most often it just appears out of nowhere. Unhelpfully, it's also often loudest when you're tired or stressed. There is no cure, but sometimes people find low-level background noise helps distract from the constant ringing.

Eyes

Have your eyes examined every year or so. Glaucoma, cataracts and macular degeneration can all be treated if detected early. What's more, a diet rich in zinc, vitamins C and E, and omega-3 fatty acids can help prevent cataracts and age-related macular degeneration.

Diabetics should be particularly vigilant, because high blood sugar can damage the blood vessels in the retina.

Older people tend to have reduced night vision, so you may find it more difficult driving after dark ... in which case, it's probably too late for carrots! Take a taxi instead.

Feet

As we get older, the skin on our feet becomes dry, cracked and calloused, and our nails grow thicker. A podiatrist can therefore be your best friend. However, if you'd rather care for your feet yourself, you can give them a good soak in a bucket of warm water with a couple of glugs of olive oil. Works wonders!

A battery-powered foot-sander is also a handy tool to have. It will deal with dry, cracked skin in no time. Just be careful to follow the directions!

And remember to include your feet in your daily moisturising routine. They will thank you for it. Tea tree oil is great for any nail fungal problems you may have.

Teeth

Healthy teeth = a healthy body. Oral health plays a critical role in our overall health and well-being. If a person is suffering from cavities or abscesses or other dental-health problems, that has a knock-on effect. Gum disease, in particular, has an immediate impact on your gut health. It's no fun being constantly in pain and rundown.

Usually, there's a dental treatment that can help, but here in New Zealand many people don't get the care they need because of the cost. A recent study showed that 40 per cent of us avoided going to the dentist because of the high expense involved, prompting a campaign for free universal dental care. Who knows how likely that really is, but at the very least I believe better care needs to be more easily and freely available for those who need it. Currently in New Zealand, dental care is free until the age of 18, and those in the most dire need may be able to access financial support via Work and Income New Zealand (WINZ), but that's clearly not enough. Too many of us, especially as we get older, are missing out on vital oral healthcare simply because of the price tag. If you're struggling with the cost of a treatment it may help to talk to your dentist about a payment plan.

There are a few things it's important to keep on top of when it comes to your teeth.

- **Get regular dental check-ups.** Ideally this should be done annually. If money is short, you may simply have to go longer between check-ups.
- **Brush your teeth twice a day** with a toothpaste containing fluoride, which will help to protect your teeth and prevent tooth decay.
- **Floss at least once a day.**
- **If you wear dentures, make sure to clean them thoroughly every day**, and soak them overnight in dental solution.

If this all sounds super basic, that's because it is! But so many of us put off the basics until they become a problem.

Yes, we are high maintenance as we age! But taking time to look after that precious body of ours will pay off a thousandfold down the track.

7

THE LONG GOODBYE
Dementia

*'When people hear the word "dementia" they forget
there's a beginning and automatically think of the end.
There's so much life still to be lived, albeit differently
and with lots of support.'*

—Wendy Mitchell, 'Wendy Mitchell on life with dementia',
Age UK

The two greatest fears I have as I age are losing my husband and losing my mind. It's the elephant in the room, isn't it? We all fear losing our capacity to think and understand, to speak coherently and function as an adult.

What's more, most of us have experienced dementia in someone close to us. Both my mother and my mother-in-law died with dementia (not from it), and it certainly made their final years distressing for them and all those who loved them.

We watched as they slowly became disoriented and confused. It was heartbreaking to see the anxiety and bewilderment in their eyes. Nothing seemed to make sense. It is heartbreaking, too, to have to essentially parent your parent.

The term dementia is, according to Alzheimers New Zealand, a catch-all used to describe a group of symptoms that affect how well our brains work. There are many causes of dementia, but the most common is Alzheimer's disease. Generally, symptoms include changes in memory, thinking, behaviour, personality and emotions. However, symptoms are unique to each person, and depend on the area of the brain affected. As dementia progresses, it will eventually start to affect a person's ability to do everyday things like getting dressed or having a shower. Dementia isn't a normal part of the ageing process, but the risk of getting it increases as we get older. It's also on the rise in New Zealand.

It may come as some comfort to know there are things that can be done to help those who develop dementia to continue to live well, and compassion can go a long way towards helping both you and them cope. There's a quote from Joanne Koenig Coste, from her book *Learning to Speak Alzheimer's*, that I particularly love:

I am seeking,
I am not lost.
I am forgetful,
I am not gone.

In other words, your loved one will be different and will need patience and tolerance, but they are still your loved one and you can still find joy with each other.

With my mum, simple routines seemed to work best. Mum used to love coming with us to our bach in the Coromandel. It was her happy place. She would sit in the sun on the verandah, her feet perched gently on the back of our big Rhodesian ridgeback, soaking in the sound of birdsong and gazing at the little bay shimmering in the distance. We would make a special effort to take her there regularly – until she suddenly began to get incredibly anxious whenever we left Auckland, that is.

By that point, she needed to be around familiar things, with her familiar routine. Our rather chaotic household was too much for her. She became agitated and irritable. Her once-sparkling conversation became stilted and unfiltered. One day she looked at me, squinting critically. 'When did you get so old?' she said. It was not what I needed to hear at the time, just entering my fifties and thinking I wasn't doing too badly on the wrinkle front! People in later-stage dementia begin to lose their inhibitions and are apt to make loud comments about other people, often in the supermarket. 'Look at that enormous woman,' Mum bellowed at me one day. 'Why would you let yourself get that fat?'

One particularly awful incident occurred when Mum had to spend a few days in hospital. A man in the same ward, also suffering from dementia, got up in the middle of the night and peed all over her bed. Poor man, he was oblivious to what he was doing, but it gave my darling mum a terrible fright. We were horrified, but these sorts of things do happen with dementia.

So it is inevitably top of mind when I think about my own future. Am I at risk of developing dementia? I can certainly be forgetful, more so lately, and have been known to leave the gas hob on more than once. The other day I came home to find firefighters surrounding the house and smoke drifting through the kitchen – someone had left a plastic spatula on a hot pan and it had melted, releasing toxic fumes. It wasn't my fault that time, but it could so easily have been. I also forget people's names. I sometimes drive to the end of the road and then realise I've forgotten where I'm going. Is this the beginning of something sinister? I wonder.

'Relax,' I'm told. 'It's a product of a frenetic life! It's normal to forget things over time. Names are lost, you're not as quick to find the right word. If you're worried about your memory, it's a good sign!'

But still, I do worry.

Is dementia genetic? The experts tell me genes only account for around a seven per cent risk of developing dementia. They say if you live a healthy, active lifestyle, that will lessen the risk, even if you have a high genetic risk. Activity that is cognitively challenging for half an hour at least five days a week is profoundly protective. Take up ballroom-dancing, kapa haka, anything that stimulates the brain to think creatively and across both hemispheres.

Neuroscientists like the University of Auckland's Sir Richard Faull ONZM are working on ways to identify genes that supress or change the genes that give you a predisposition for dementia. They are also working on early detection, so that doctors can begin treatment before the tau and amyloid proteins – which emerging evidence suggests have a big part to play in the onset of Alzheimer's – begin to kill off brain cells.

The latest report from Alzheimers New Zealand, prepared by researchers at Auckland University, shows that dementia constitutes a major and still rapidly growing problem for New Zealand. It has multiple impacts and costs for individuals, for society, for the health system and for the economy. The report indicates that nearly three per cent of all New Zealanders will have dementia by 2050, including more than ten per cent of our over-65 population. That's a 240 per cent increase in the next 30 years. Sobering statistics.

According to the University of Auckland's Ngaire Kerse, 'Dementia is not happening to Māori any more than non-Māori. Even though many Māori have endured a lifetime of deprivation and discrimination, which has impacted their entire life ... they are extremely resilient in cognition.' Why? Some researchers believe this may be because of the richness of Māori culture. For instance, for those who speak te reo, being bilingual is good for the brain. With something like kapa haka, the moves are complicated and there's a lot to remember – and that, too, preserves cognition.

Reducing your risk

Here's the thing. There are a number of ways you can reduce your risk of dementia. In fact, almost 40 per cent of dementia cases in New Zealand can be prevented or delayed.

- **Look after your heart.** According to Richard Faull, 'What's good for the heart is good for the brain.' As well as increasing the risk of heart attacks and strokes, things like high cholesterol, high blood pressure, diabetes and obesity also increase the risk of dementia. This is because they reduce the flow of blood to the brain. Each time your heart pumps, it sends about 25 per cent of the body's blood to the brain.

- **Midlife matters.** Incremental changes begin decades earlier. Take care of yourself in your forties and fifties. If you've already crossed that hurdle, it's never too late. Take care of yourself now!

- **Throw away those cigarettes.** Not only are they hazardous to your lungs (as well as your budget), they are strongly linked to an increased risk of dementia.

- **Limit your alcohol intake.** Alcohol mounts a direct attack on the brain cells, and with excessive drinking the brain actually shrinks. Alcohol also affects the heart, limiting the supply of blood to the brain. The good news, though, is that if you stop drinking, the damage may be partly reversible. Some function can return.

- **Eat well.** Obesity is a key risk factor for developing dementia. The current advice is seven servings of fruit and vegetables per day. (See pages 30–35 for more information on the kinds of foods to zero in on.) Scientists now know that what you ate in your childhood is important for brain health as you age. Astonishingly, American research shows women with longer legs have a reduced risk of Alzheimer's.

For every 2.5 centimetres of increase in leg length, the risk reduced by 16 per cent! In men, only arm length seemed to matter – for every 2.5 centimetres of increased length, there was a six per cent decrease in dementia. Scientists speculate that arm and leg length may relate to poor nutrition in childhood.

- **Exercise.** Do anything from brisk walking to paddle-boarding to tai chi four or five times a week to keep the heart pumping, the blood vessels strong and the blood flowing, sending nutrients flushing through the brain. If it makes you huff and puff, all the better! Walk the dog with a friend. You'll chat while you walk, and that's guaranteed to get your heart rate up.

- **Make time for friends and family.** Socialising stimulates the brain and can reduce cardiovascular disease. It lowers stress levels. With stress comes an increase in cortisol, and too much cortisol tends to eat away at your brain cells. What's more, research shows that interacting with others slows the progression of dementia. If you stay at home with a stressed carer, the chances are you will speed up the decline.

- **Get a hearing check.** Around 80 per cent of people with dementia have hearing loss, so if you're missing parts of conversations or having to turn the telly up, go and get a hearing check. If you need a hearing aid, getting one will reduce your risk.

- **Build the brain.** Learn a language. Play a musical instrument. Do Wordle or crosswords or sudoku.

Play chess or bridge or memory games. Get the grandchildren to play, too, if you have them. Focus on the can-do. Keep the old grey matter active!

Warning signs

If you're worried that either you or someone you love may be developing dementia, there are some classic warning signs to look out for:

- **Recent memory loss, or forgetting recent events.** People with early dementia begin to forget their grandchildren's names. They write lists and leave notes around the house.
- **Difficulty performing regular tasks.** A person with dementia may have trouble finding their way home from their favourite café or driving a regular route.
- **Problems with language.** We all find ourselves grasping for words at times, but people with dementia find it difficult to keep track of conversations or even to begin one.
- **Confusion about the time of day.** People with dementia can easily lose track of time and what it is they're supposed to be doing. For this reason it's good to try to keep to a routine.
- **Decreased or poor judgement.** Bad decisions may be made, for instance around things like paying bills or giving presents.
- **Lack of attention to basic grooming.** A person may not notice stains on their clothes, or may forget to shower or brush their hair.

- **Problems with abstract thinking.** People with dementia may have trouble figuring out how to use numbers, or even what they are.
- **Misplacing things.** Household objects may appear in odd places: the car keys in the fridge, shoes in the oven and so on.
- **Changes in mood and behaviour.** Mood swings can become the norm, especially extreme swings from calm to anger, or happy to tears.
- **Loss of initiative.** While we all lose the will to tackle things on our to-do list from time to time, people with dementia may no longer want to do things they used to enjoy, like tending the garden, exercising or socialising.
- **Changes in personality.** We can all get a little grumpy with age. Some of us even get cranky and cantankerous. And some get, as my dad used to say, 'shitty-livered'! But dementia sufferers may suddenly have a major problem with something that never previously bothered them.

Diagnosis

Be vigilant. If you spot any of these warning signs, don't wait. Go and see your GP.

Don't be afraid. Yet again, knowledge is power. Ignorance is *not* bliss. An early diagnosis will give you time to understand the condition fully, to plan and to get your affairs in order. It will also allow you to make the most of your time. What's more, there are treatments out there that can stall or delay the decline.

More generally, make sure you let your GP know if you have a family history of dementia. Take a memory test with your GP every few years. This test usually takes around five minutes, and assesses skills like reading, writing, orientation (which often involves simply asking the patient's full name, current location and the date) and short-term memory.

There are several different types of dementia. The main ones are as follows:

- **Alzheimer's** affects 50 to 70 per cent of all those with dementia, and is caused by plaques and tangles in the brain. Early on, you will notice memory and learning problems. Around 80 per cent of sufferers develop psychological and behavioural problems, such as depression and apathy. In the mid-stage, psychosis is common, as well as irritability, agitation and wandering. Late-stage Alzheimer's patients may experience incontinence and difficulty walking and swallowing.
- **Vascular dementia** is caused by damage to the vessels supplying blood to the brain. It causes a gradual decline in attention, decision-making, memory, learning, language and social behaviour. It tends to attack the prefrontal cortex – the part of the brain responsible for judgement, planning and decision-making.
- **Lewy body dementia** occurs when abnormal clumps of proteins called Lewy bodies form on the brain's cortex and destroy nerve cells. Those with Lewy body dementia may display Parkinson's type symptoms, such as shaking,

muscle rigidity or stiffness, slow movements or shuffling, quiet speech and reduced facial expression.

- **Frontotemporal dementia** affects the frontal and/or temporal lobes of the brain. The frontal lobe manages our thinking, emotions, personality, judgement and self-control. It also plays a part in muscle control, movement and memory storage. The temporal lobes are part of our sensory processing system – they're important in hearing, understanding language, and storing and retrieving memories. If a person's frontal lobes are affected, they may have trouble with motivation, organisation and planning, and behaving in a socially appropriate way. If the temporal lobes are affected, they may have difficulty speaking and possibly understanding language. Symptoms can begin as early as 50.

A diagnosis of dementia is not a death sentence. It is a disability, just like any other. Life can go on, and better yet it can be rewarding and wonderful for many years. There are new medications coming into the field all the time. There are ways to slow the progression of the disease. Early detection, though, makes all the difference.

In an interview with Age UK, Wendy Mitchell shared her personal experience of living with dementia. She vividly recalled the day she was diagnosed with young-onset Alzheimer's at the age of 58. 'The consultant had a sad look on her face, gave me a handshake and said, "Goodbye – there's nothing we can do,"' Mitchell said. 'Imagine the psychological impact of being told that! I'm not downplaying it's a bummer of a diagnosis, but if she'd instead said something like, "I'm afraid it is dementia, but think of it as the start of a different life," my mindset would have been so different when I left her office.'

A self-described glass-half-full person, Mitchell vowed to outwit the disease for as long as she could. 'I like to think of a diagnosis as the beginning of a different life,' she said. 'One of adapting and support, and not one you'd have imagined whatsoever, but the start of a new life rather than the end of life.'

In her 2018 memoir *Somebody I Used to Know*, Mitchell talks about some of the simple things she does to jog her memory. Things like naming household rooms and large items with Post-It notes, and creating a 'memory room' with lines of photos on the walls. 'One row has her daughters, another the places Wendy lived, a third her favourite views – the Lake District and Blackpool Beach,' author Meik Wiking wrote of this room in his book *The Art of Making Memories*. He quotes Wendy: 'I sit on the edge of the bed in front of them [the photos], feeling that same sense of calm and happiness. When the memories have emptied on the inside, they'll still be here on the outside – a constant reminder, a feeling of happier times.'

A diagnosis of dementia might be devastating and frightening, but as Wendy Mitchell shows, it does not mean there is no hope. Life has changed, but it can still be meaningful and contain happiness.

Find the potential

I can't think of a better illustration of how people with dementia should be treated than the wonderful New Zealand film *Hip*

Hop-eration, which tells the heartwarming story of a hip-hop dance group for people aged over 65.

When Billie Jordan first moved to Waiheke Island in her early forties she was lonely and isolated and afraid. She noticed a number of her elderly neighbours appeared to feel the same way, so she decided to do something about it. She drove around the island in her van, asking anyone who looked over 65 whether they'd like to join a hip-hop group. Maybe it's a Waiheke thing – something about embracing the fun side of life – but, amazingly, the people she approached didn't think she was a lunatic! Jordan didn't know anything about hip-hop, but she taught herself a few moves by watching YouTube videos, and passed those moves on to her recruits. Thus the Hip Hop-eration crew was formed.

There were 22 members, ranging in age from 68 to 96. Five had dementia, one was blind, six were deaf, four used mobility aids, most had had a hip replacement and they all had arthritis. The thing was, nobody expected anything of them, but as Jordan said, that's 'so demoralising' – so she set them an audacious goal to make it to the World Hip Hop Championships in Las Vegas. She treated her dancers as equals, had high expectations of them and never let their age or state of mind be an excuse. 'Instead of stifling older people's abilities,' she said, 'we should be doing everything we can to maximise their potential.'

People with dementia have potential. They want and need to be treated like capable human beings. For her dancers with dementia, Jordan focused particularly on muscle memory, because it's stronger, she says, than brain memory. Her elderly crew began to look more alive. They stopped looking backwards and looked towards the future. Their doctors said they were fitter and happier than they'd been in years. And yes, they did make it to Las Vegas – and, what's more, they were sensational!

It's encouraging to know that 60 per cent of dementia is modifiable. Yet services to help people with dementia are clearly not able to keep up with the increasing demand. By 2050, ten per cent of all superannuitants will have dementia. Age Concern's former CEO Stephanie Clare told me it's time for better management methods. 'Don't lock them up,' she pleads. 'It's important for people with dementia to mix with a range of age groups.'

In most care homes, intergenerational relationships rely on staff and relatives to take people out. But some homes have children coming in to interact with the residents. One resident began sketching the children. No one knew he was an artist. It was a win–win. The residents were more engaged with what was going on around them. The levels of agitation, aggression and dementia dropped, they were calmer, and the children's attitudes to older people changed.

There are several key things you can do to help a loved one with dementia find joy and realise their potential:

- **Encourage them to do things they've always enjoyed.**
  Music, crafts, teaching … Make these things possible.
  Remember what it was they loved to do and what they were
  interested in, and focus on those things.
- **Get dancing and singing!** Music and singing can be
  great stimulators for the brain, and the ability to sing
  and appreciate music is often preserved even into late

dementia. Use the soundtrack of their lives. My mum used to love listening to Tchaikovsky's *Swan Lake*. It reminded her of her days as a ballet dancer. We'd play it over and over, as well as the songs from old musicals like *South Pacific* and *Gigi* that she loved to sing along to with Dad.

- **Activity helps.** Do sit–stand exercises to help prevent falls and work on lower leg strength and balance. If you notice an increase in restlessness or agitation in the late afternoon (often known as 'sundowning' and more common in the later stages of dementia), some gentle activity around this time can help, such as a stroll in the outdoors or doing some light exercise while listening to music.

- **Try fidget bags.** These can be useful as the dementia progresses. Fill them with items that will stimulate memories. Add different textures and shapes. Mum's included a piece of lace from her wedding dress, some velvet, a little box, some shells from the beach she loved, and of course photos of her family.

- **Offer snacks regularly.** Dementia often causes a loss of appetite. When you eat, do it together, as that encourages people to eat more. Put vegetables in a smoothie.

- **Make the loo stand out.** Make it a different colour so there's no confusion about which whiteware to use! In addition, put a picture of the loo on the door of the bathroom.

- **Beware of UTIs.** Undetected, urinary tract infections can cause an increase in agitation and aggression. A good indicator is smell – the urine will smell quite pungent.

- **Pull-ups are best.** While incontinence diapers are good, the ones that pull up just like underwear are best.
- **Connect to childhood.** People with dementia often want to retreat into their childhood. We found giving Mum a life-sized baby doll settled her and gave her focus.
- **Seek peer support.** According to Wendy Mitchell, the biggest support for her was hearing others say, 'That happened to me.' As she says, 'You can feel very alone with a diagnosis of dementia, especially if you don't know anyone else who has it, but listening to and laughing with other people with dementia is wonderful.'

Caring

Caring for a loved one with dementia can be hard. It is a huge responsibility, and it is exhausting and relentless. The journey begins slowly, with commitment, love and devotion, but as the years wear on and the symptoms begin to increase in severity, it becomes harder and harder.

Collectively, New Zealand whānau are slogging through a million hours of unpaid caring a week for their relatives living with dementia. This is particularly pronounced in Pasifika cultures, where service to your family and your wider community is simply a given. In many cases, it's grandchildren who are the caregivers. Some have to give up their schooling to care for elderly relatives, while their parents work to make ends meet. Looking after your elders is more than a duty in Pasifika cultures, however. It's seen as a blessing. That's not to say it's easy, though. Far from it.

Dementia support services are already lacking, but this is even more pronounced for communities with access and cultural issues to overcome. It's an inequity of care and lack of culturally competent services that Alzheimers New Zealand says is unacceptable – especially when you consider that dementia rates in Māori, Pasifika and Asian communities are set to more than double by 2050.

If you do find yourself caring for a loved one with dementia, there are a few things it can help to know:

- **Try to keep calm and speak gently.** People with dementia become sensitive to tone, and they will sense your impatience. They need to feel loved.
- **Try not to stand over them.** Instead, speak to them on the same level, making eye contact.
- **Don't sweat the small stuff.** If a person with dementia says it's Thursday, says Richard Faull, then it's Thursday. Don't keep correcting them, even if it is, in fact, Wednesday. It doesn't matter. Better to ignore it and not antagonise the brain. Just concentrate on helping them to do the things they can do.

People with dementia often have trouble sleeping, and may wake several times in the night and become agitated. They may wander around the house, or even decide to take themselves off for a walk outside. As a result, you'll find yourself missing out on sleep, too. You may simply need to stay awake so you can keep an eye on your charge, or you may find yourself spending precious hours settling them back into bed.

As well as taking an emotional toll, being a caregiver is also often physically draining. For instance, you may need a hoist to lift a person in and out of bed. The inevitable exhaustion you experience may leave you feeling hopeless and unable to cope.

It's OK – in fact, it's right – to ask for help. Many rest homes and hospitals offer respite care so you can take time out from your 24-hour caring role and let someone else do the heavy lifting for a while. It's difficult to ask for help. It might be the first time you've ever had to do it. But asking for help will make you a better carer in the end.

Hollywood star Bruce Willis has a list of film credits as long as your arm, but he's probably best known for his role as John McClane in the *Die Hard* movies. In March 2022, his family announced that he had been diagnosed with frontotemporal dementia. His wife, Emma Hemmings Willis, has been determined to do her very best to support him, and after he was approached during a rare visit to a café with friends, she posted a plea to social media asking paparazzi to give him space. Hemmings Willis talked about how stressful it is getting a person with dementia out into the world and navigating it safely, and noted that she has gained enormous strength from the support of dementia-care consultant Teepa Snow. An occupational therapist with 40 years of clinical practice, Snow's key message for carers is to become a 'care partner', not a 'care giver'. Work together; don't try to push care onto your loved one. Snow advises carers to start by realising they are on a journey – a long journey. 'Try not to do the Lone Ranger thing,' she says. 'You'll run out of gas.' She advises doing your research: 'There are lots of things out there to help you. Find out about them.' And most importantly, 'Learn the art of letting it go. Take a moment, breathe and learn.'

You can learn more about Snow's Positive Approach to Care on her website (teepasnow.com), and there are a few other online resources you might also turn to for help.

- The **Dementia New Zealand** website (dementia.nz) offers information, resources and support for people with dementia and their loved ones.
- The **Alzheimers New Zealand** website (alzheimers. org.nz) provides local support contact info and further information about dementia.
- **Age Concern New Zealand/He Manaakitanga Kaumātua Aotearoa** (ageconcern.org.nz) is a charity dedicated to people over 65, their friends and whānau. They promote dignity, well-being, equity and respect, and provide information and support services.

Caregivers have often told me they feel invisible in the community, especially since many of them are holding down jobs as well. One woman who was caring for her mother at home told researchers she felt she had to keep quiet about it, because she felt it 'set a bad example to her workers if she took time away from work to take her mother to a doctor's appointment'. How sad is that?

Nearly half a million New Zealanders provide unpaid care for people with disability, and 35 per cent of those carers are over 55. Carers need to feel supported by the whole of society, not abandoned by it.

I want to give the last word in this chapter to Billie Jordan: 'There is no shame in having dementia. It is not a deal-breaker for living a fulfilling, happy, rewarding life, as long as you've got good people around you and courage.'

PART 2

Well-being

8

IT TAKES TWO
Relationships

'Count your life by smiles, not tears.
Count your age by friends, not years.'
—Author unknown

W hen Laurence Reynolds died at the age of 107 in July 2022, he was New Zealand's oldest man. 'He always chose to live, and to live fully,' his son Roger told the *New Zealand Herald*. 'Even in his final days, he hoisted himself up to a sitting position and I heard him call out, "I think I need a pacemaker!"'

After an early brush with death at the age of 28, Laurence gained what his son called a 'dogged determination to live' and went on to become one of our country's coronary care pioneers. As well as establishing the first coronary care unit and the first cardiac rehabilitation unit in New Zealand, he was also the first to advocate for the early mobilisation of heart patients in order to avoid clotting.

Laurence was always matter of fact about his own health problems, seeing them as something to be dealt with rather than dwelt on. He walked every day until he was 106, and when asked the secret to his longevity, his son said it was 'his relationship with our mum'. Laurence was married to Claire for 75 years – she died just before him in the same year, at the age of 95 – and the two of them lived their lives 'looking forward and without regret', their son said.

Time and again, gerontologists will tell you that social connection – having people you care about and who care about you – is one of the most important keys to ageing well. (That, and a positive attitude – more on that later.) Case in point: emeritus professor Dame Peggy Koopman-Boyden told me, 'Social connectedness is the most important critical issue facing older people. Having a number of friends who are concerned about you – people who have that in their lives will live longer. Connecting and getting out and about in the world is important, rather than making your world the kitchen, the garden, the house.'

Take the Study of Adult Development. It is, as far as we know, the world's longest study of human life that's ever been done. Based at Harvard Medical School and Massachusetts General Hospital, it's been going for 85 years and has covered three generations: grandparents, parents and children. By now, the researchers have studied over 2000 people altogether; every two years they question participants about their lives, peruse their medical records, scan their brains, take their blood and talk to their spouses and their children.

So what has this huge study found? What is it that contributes to our health and well-being as we age? 'There were two big items over 85 years,' the study's fourth director, Robert Waldinger, told McKinsey & Company in 2023. 'One is taking care of our health.' Good news! We've already covered that in Part 1 of this book.

'The part that surprised us,' Waldinger went on, 'was that the people who were happiest, who stayed healthiest as they grew old, and who lived the longest were the people who had the warmest connections with other people.'

Those who were happiest at 50, the study found, were healthiest at 80. And those who were happiest in retirement were the people who nurtured relationships with family, friends and their community. They tended to replace screen-time with people time, taking long walks together, going on date nights. As *The Harvard Gazette* summed it up, 'Close relationships, more than money or fame, are what keep people happy throughout their lives … Those ties protect people from life's discontents, help to delay mental and physical decline, and are better predictors of long and happy lives than social class, IQ, or even genes.'

'There's nothing new in the idea that good relationships are good for us,' I hear you say. And yet it seems we have taken our eye off the ball in this regard. More and more of us are entering older age alone. The rate of divorce is higher than it's ever been, and that's hitting men particularly hard because they tend to have smaller social networks and retirement can be a lonely time for them. Too often, we seem to prize external success – in the form of money, social status, achievements or material trappings – over our relationships with our loved ones.

Waldinger reckons that's simply because we're human. We want the quick fix. Relationships are messy and complicated. They're not glamorous. They require lifelong hard work. But they are also the key to a happy and healthy life. We instinctively know this, yet we insist on pursuing all those material trappings with a zeal that defies logic!

According to Waldinger, there are three significant things the study has highlighted about the importance of relationships:

1. **Social connection is really good for us.** Good relationships keep us happier and healthier – they lead to an increase in the feel-good hormone oxytocin, lower stress and reduce inflammation. Even seemingly inconsequential chats with your local barista or supermarket checkout operator can give you little hits of oxytocin during the day!

2. **Quality trumps quantity.** It's not being in a committed relationship or the number of friends you have that matters so much as the quality of those relationships.

3. **Your relationships can affect how you deal with pain.** Those who suffer physical pain and are in happy relationships are still able to maintain a happy mood, despite their pain. However, for those in unhappy relationships, the physical pain is magnified and reflects in their mood.

Romance

In Mitch Albom's bestselling memoir *Tuesdays with Morrie*, his old professor recounts the things he knows to be true about love and marriage. For an enduring and happy marriage, he tells Albom, you need mutual respect, tolerance, communication, common values and a belief in the importance of marriage.

I love that. Those five key ingredients really resonate with me, and they can equally be applied to friendships. *Tuesdays with Morrie* is one of my bibles – it's about a series of visits Albom made to his old sociology professor, Morrie Schwartz, while Morrie was dying of ALS, a progressive nervous system disease. The book contains all kinds of pearls of wisdom. Seek it out if you haven't read it. I guarantee it will make you think about your life.

When it comes to marriages or partnerships in particular, the Harvard study found a strong correlation between the state of your relationship at 50 and the way you will age at 80. Those who were in a loving, mutually happy relationship at 50 were the healthiest at 80. So it seems that really was Laurence Reynolds's secret!

Don't worry, no one is suggesting your relationships have to be perfectly lovey-dovey 100 per cent of the time. Bickering is OK. (Our grandchildren have taken to pointing out our bickering, so Chris and I must do it a bit. I would call it constructive discussion!) Waldinger notes that many octogenarian couples do it day in day out. He says it's fine so long as you can rely on each other. Good relationships are protective for the brain, and a happy marriage is extremely protective. At the same time, however, living in conflict is going to be bad for your health – worse, in fact, than experiencing a divorce.

Always an active man, Doug Bullick first began having trouble with his legs in his mid-nineties. For the last few years of his life, he used a Zimmer frame and a walking stick to negotiate his two-storey home. He also slept downstairs, while his wife of 73 years, May (also in her nineties), slept upstairs. Doug had always taken May her cup of tea in the mornings, and he wasn't one to let a couple of dodgy legs set him back. He had a second handrail installed on the stairway so he could grasp both sides, and he tied a thermos of tea around his neck to get her cuppa upstairs. Such was his devotion to the love of his life.

Before he died in 2022 at the age of 101, Doug said that the two tools that had helped him live a happy life were compromise and helping others. 'You can't always win,' he said. 'We were brought up to help people when we can and be prepared to compromise.'

His advice for the younger generation? 'Think of other people and look after your neighbour.'

Now that's a good set of footprints to follow!

Loneliness

Our need for social connection is as fundamental to us as our need to eat. Loneliness, by contrast, is toxic.

It has a direct physical impact. Those who are isolated are, unsurprisingly, less happy, but also their health declines more rapidly in midlife and they generally die earlier. In fact, one study from Brigham Young University showed loneliness is more deadly than obesity, and that lacking social connection can be more dangerous than smoking 15 cigarettes a day!

The physical toll of loneliness is sobering. Research has shown lonely people have more trouble climbing stairs and bathing themselves. Loneliness also causes neural responses in the brain similar to those caused by hunger. It causes stress, too, and in the long term leads to a rise in cortisol. High cortisol levels, as mentioned earlier, are linked to higher levels of inflammation in the body, which in turn damages blood vessels and other tissues and can lead to an increased risk of heart disease, joint pain, depression and obesity.

Loneliness is a global challenge. The UK and Japan take it so seriously that both have appointed government ministers for loneliness, tasked with the job of building connections between people. Here in New Zealand, Age Concern reports that more than ten per cent of over-75s are lonely all, most or some of the time. One Otago University study found that just over 20 per cent of frail elderly people were lonely. (People who are frail usually have a combination of symptoms that include unintentional weight loss, muscle loss and weakness, and a feeling of fatigue. For more information, see pages 55–57.)

Asian respondents in the study were most likely to be lonely – quite possibly, researchers suggested, because many had come to New Zealand to support their children, who were studying here, but had little English and found it difficult to fit in. Pasifika people were the least likely to experience loneliness, largely because of their extended-family support systems.

As noted earlier, health and well-being in te ao Māori is seen collectively, wrapped up in the community. A strong sense of who you are and where you fit in is key, as is the spiritual dimension.

Karakia or prayer are fundamentally important. Interestingly, according to one social worker, Māori are actually more likely to report being lonely, whereas Pākehā just 'expect' to be lonely.

There is a lot of embarrassment and shame around loneliness, and this prevents people from asking for help. They don't want to be a burden. Many think it's their own fault, or that admitting how they feel would reflect poorly on the whānau who care for them.

Early childhood experiences can also have an impact on whether or not we suffer from loneliness. Parental conflict, bullying and poverty can all make us less resilient as adults, and therefore more insecure and prone to becoming lonely. People who have difficulty regulating their emotions or who become easily 'rattled' also have an increased risk of loneliness.

Reaching out

When I first started my role on the nightly TV news, I didn't think much about what it would entail outside of work. I was just living in the moment, rejoicing in the job. But, bit by bit, I gained an increasingly public profile. I lost my anonymity. It was anathema to a shy person like me.

You don't realise how precious anonymity is until it's gone. I became more and more self-conscious, more worried about what people thought of me. Did I measure up? Was I good enough? Those thoughts continue to plague me, especially when I'm about to try something new. It's a lonely place to be.

Experiencing loneliness is a vicious cycle. Lonely people are more apprehensive about social situations, and pick up on perceived social-rejection cues too quickly. They may misread those cues, and believe people are thinking negative things about them when the opposite is true.

One thing about loneliness is that it resides within. You can be lonely even when you're surrounded by people. I have certainly felt that from time to time. So has interviewee Pam. Now in her seventies, she says she often feels invisible at family gatherings. 'It's almost as if the rest of the family are talking a different language,' she says. She can't help feeling, while her family are busy chatting around her, that she's being overlooked.

Another thing about loneliness is that it's not the same as being alone. Some people, myself included, are profoundly happy in their own company. Alone time is good. It can help you reconnect with yourself. Too much of it, though, is not good. We are not created to be alone all the time. We are social beings. The more connected we are, the more we thrive.

We're all different. If you're introverted, it's more difficult to initiate connections with others; extroverts, though, feed off social contact. The question to ask yourself is, 'Am I as connected to others as I want to be?'

Gerontologist Dame Peggy Koopman-Boyden says, 'Societal isolation is a private matter. It behoves the rest of us to scoop up people who are alone.' We can all do our bit to address loneliness, even if we're lonely ourselves. For instance, if you're at a gathering and you notice someone sitting alone, Koopman-Boyden suggests you go and sit beside them. Strike up a conversation. If we, as a society, invest in ways to better support social connection and reduce loneliness, I suspect it would save us a lot of money and heartache down the track.

There are some wonderfully positive things that communities can do to help older people who are feeling isolated. Eastern Bay Villages/ Te Kokoru Manaakitanga is a group of locals in the Eastern Bay of Plenty who want to age well in their own homes and communities, and actively encourage others to do the same. They have a specific focus on working together to reduce isolation and vulnerability among seniors. 'We're just a bunch of old people helping each other stay out of the rest home, and we have innovative ways to do that,' coordinator Ruth Gerzon told me. Of course, they're much more than that. Ruth has a rich background in community development and has enabled the group to share skills and knowledge to scaffold each other and advocate for others.

For instance, they've set up a 'home share' scheme, where people in their fifties or sixties live in an older person's house rent-free in return for ten hours a week of company. The relationship is one of companionship, rather than providing caring tasks like showering or meals. 'Everything we do is about relationships,' Gerzon says. 'The health benefits are clear. An over-70-year-old with one new younger friend can live an extra two years. It's better than giving up smoking!'

When trying to address feelings of loneliness, it's important to figure out why you're feeling ignored, disconnected and isolated. It's vital that you break the mental cycle of believing you're not worthy of friendship. Sometimes, those feelings sneak up on you before you know it. Sometimes, they're born out of tragedy.

As we age, we will inevitably lose some of our closest friends, those with whom we can share our most intimate thoughts. When you go way back with someone, they really know you. They understand what makes you who you are, and they are forgiving of your foibles. My mate Deb and I first became friends in primary school. We went to boarding school together, traversed all those teenage rites of passage, and shared all of life's ups and downs. She and her husband, Paul, lived just around the corner, which was great because Deb was a spectacular cook and threw legendary parties. We were looking forward to growing old together. So, when Deb called me one day out of the blue to tell me she had just been diagnosed with motor neurone disease, I was heartbroken.

Deb was a nurse. She knew what she was in for. Motor neurone disease leaves you trapped inside your body. The nerve cells that control the muscles waste away, taking with them the ability to move, speak, swallow and ultimately breathe. She might last a year or maybe four. Her decline was mercifully swift, but it was dreadful to watch. Those of us in her support crew did our best to keep her laughing and to lighten the load on her wonderful husband, who gave up his job to take on her full-time care.

Deb had a wicked sense of humour, and when the disease took her voice she would type outrageous things on her iPad for our amusement. We took her out for walks in her wheelchair, we went to lunch, she watched while we weeded her garden and, in the process, those of us in her support crew renewed old friendships ourselves. It was a painful, beautiful, deeply personal, intimate time. Paul is often asked how he coped during those terrible months, and his answer is always, 'Friendship. Without friends I would have ended up a patient, too.'

The loss of Deb was enormous. She will never be replaced. However, even in the most dire of circumstances, there was still comfort to be found. I still miss her.

No matter the cause, it's important to address loneliness, to try to find new friends when old ones pass away, because at its worst loneliness can cause cognitive decline, resulting in dementia. The reverse is also true: dementia can cause loneliness. And if that's not reason enough to do something about it, try this one for size: lonely people are more likely to end up in rest-home care.

When it comes to making new friends, social media is both a blessing and a curse. It can be a great way to meet people with similar interests, to find your tribe. A friend who'd just moved out of Auckland told me about a Facebook group she'd joined. It began when another woman posted a message saying she, too, was new to the area, didn't know a soul and wondered if anyone was interested in meeting for coffee and/or adventures. The group now numbers 200! They don't all meet at the same time, but they've had some great fun together.

The downside of social media, of course, is that most people only post life's greatest hits. It can look like everyone else is having a marvellous time without you, which can lead to increased loneliness. Remember, it's not like that all the time. You never know what's going on behind the façade. Don't fall into the trap of comparing yourself to what you see online. As Teddy Roosevelt was reportedly fond of saying, 'Comparison is the thief of joy.' How right he was. If you're finding that your social media feeds are making you miserable, turn them off for a bit. Take a break from them.

It's easiest to develop new friendships if you run into the same people over and over again. Share an interest or activity. Volunteer for a charity or landscape improvements in the community. Join a sports club – these will all become natural places to start a conversation.

Joining a choir is another great way to meet people and, what's more, singing is proven to lift the spirits! If you're single, it's also, Koopman-Boyden tells me, a great way to meet those of the opposite sex … As she points out, the older a woman gets, the fewer men there are.

Making friends requires effort. Try to overcome your shyness because when you push yourself, you usually end up having a good time!

I know it's all very well to say you must do something about being lonely, but it can be quite another thing to actually *do* it. Plucking up the courage to join a bridge club or a walking group or an art class may feel like a step too far, but there are several psychological approaches that can help with loneliness.

- **Cognitive behaviour therapy (CBT)** helps you understand your thoughts and feelings so you can manage your behaviour. The aim is to gain more insight into your thought processes so you can think more realistically about certain things. You can ask your GP to recommend a therapist.
- **Positive psychology** is, according to the late American psychologist Christopher Peterson, 'the scientific study

of what makes life most worth living'. It focuses on the positive things in life, including experiences like happiness and joy, and traits like gratitude and resilience. For more information, you can visit positivepsychology.com.

- **Mindfulness** can also be useful, in that the practice helps you to become aware of your thoughts so you can accept or reject them. I have also found meditation a wonderful way to centre myself and find calm within. For more on that, see pages 273–275.

Don't despair. As American author Mandy Hale wrote, 'A season of loneliness and isolation is when the caterpillar gets its wings. Remember that next time you feel alone.'

I would encourage you to screw up your courage and take the plunge to make new friends. You won't regret it.

Nurture your relationships and your friendships, and they will nurture you.

Moving

For many, retirement comes at the same time as thinking about downsizing your home or moving somewhere quieter. But moving comes with a few considerations.

People who move often find themselves more isolated. They leave their friends and family behind. Even those casual relationships with the local butcher, pharmacist and barista are little connections you have to let go. Yes, you will make new friends, but there's nothing like shared history.

And what happens if you become ill? Can you access the care you need? Will your loved ones be able to visit if the hospital is out of town? All of us hope to be fit and capable well into our retirement, but some of us will need extra care. What's more, the sort of health events that require hospital care – things like heart attacks or strokes – can occur suddenly. While the majority of us will be fine, life is a huge lottery. It's important to at least have an idea of what you're in for, should the worst happen.

University of Auckland professor Ngaire Kerse's advice is to test the waters before you make any big moves. And be careful when choosing where you go, she warns. If you love going to the opera, don't move to Kawerau!

Some decide this is the time to make the move to a retirement village, and the social aspect is often a consideration. A number of those I spoke to in researching this book agreed that, if you decide it's right for you, it's good to enter a village while you're mentally and physically able. Many said it's too late once you're in your eighties. 'If I'd had to enter on my own, I would have found it really, really hard,' says my 87-year-old friend Frances. 'It's hard when people have already formed their friend groups.' Another good time to enter a village, she adds, is when it's still in its infancy. 'At that stage, everyone's new, we're all pioneers and have that in common.'

For Pam, security was a big thing. 'Women on their own feel vulnerable out in the community. I'd been worried that when I moved into a village there'd be people knocking on the door all the time,' she said, but instead she's found 'people are respectful of others' privacy. They do care about each other, there's always someone who's happy to help you if needed.'

Gordon, who is 88, lives in a retirement village, where his beloved wife, Rosalie, is in dementia care. He is able to visit her often, and also plays a big part in the local Rotary club and is treasurer of the local University of the Third Age group. He walks 30 minutes a day, five days a week. Gordon's recipe for a healthy old age is to keep busy and positive, and he says he has a quality of life in the village that he would never have had if he'd been alone in the community. The friendships he's made there are precious. 'Growing old isn't for the faint-hearted,' he says. 'You have to make the most of your final years.'

In general, retirement villages are marketed as a 'lifestyle choice'. The ads make them look like havens for active, fit and healthy 60- to 70-year-olds, but the reality is a little different. Villages tend to attract those from their mid-seventies onwards, and a lot of those people have health issues that will interfere with an up-and-jumpin' lifestyle. However, I know from my mum and dad, my in-laws, and now both my brother and sister that they are a great option. Residents generally have all the benefits of the lifestyle, which include no maintenance or security worries, access to 24-hour nursing care should they need it, and the ability to move to a hospital on-site if necessary. Do make sure that any village you choose has a hospital attached. If you are moving in with a partner or spouse, it means that, if one of you gets sick and needs long-term care, you can still both be in the same village and close enough to be able to visit easily.

If the worst happens and I find myself without Chris and on my own, I will think seriously about moving into a village. (Of course, for his part, Chris wouldn't *dream* of going into one if the circumstances were reversed. He's busy lining up the kids and making sure they have enough bedrooms to accommodate a decrepit old bloke ... Not that he's actually discussed that with them!) As well as the benefits I've already mentioned, retirement villages can offer the companionship of like-minded people, which is especially vital given that people so often become isolated on their own in the community. Many villages also have facilities like swimming pools, bowling and croquet greens, pétanque courts, gyms, theatres, cafés, restaurants and hairdressers. And you can lock-and-leave and go on holiday without worrying about who's looking after the place. What's not to like?

There's just one thing missing: contact with young people. That is so important, and that lack is probably the biggest drawback. A number of retirement villages are actively pursuing contact with young people by partnering with their local schools. One I know of helped its neighbouring primary school to set up raised garden beds, and the village residents are teaching the children the finer points of vegetable growing. In return, the kids are learning to value the knowledge of their elderly neighbours. My little granddaughters' primary school partnered up with the local retirement village to learn about what life was like when the older people were young. They exchanged letters and visited each other at the village. It was such a simple thing to do, yet it sparked real friendships. In other towns, organisations like Plunket may even partner with villages to arrange for new parents to visit with their babies. What joy that would bring! Relationships are forged and stories told.

As I navigate this period of evolution (I did say not to mention the R-word!), I am trying to take George Vaillant's advice, and Gordon's, too. To live each day in the moment. To try to, as Eric Idle would sing, 'always look on the bright side of life'. To rejoice in family and friends. To look outside myself and to find a purpose in helping others. To see the glass as half full.

9

GRANDPARENTING 101
Looking after kids

*'There are only two lasting bequests we can hope
to give our children. One of these is roots,
the other, wings.'*
—Author unknown

I adored my gran. She was four foot nine and cuddly, a pair of wire-framed specs perched jauntily on the end of her nose. She smiled a lot.

Gran lived in a little blue fibrolite bach she dubbed 'Hi Noon'. It was nestled at the foot of the sandhills on Waikanae Beach, and I often stayed with her in the holidays. I am the youngest in my family – my brother and sister are ten and twelve years older than me, respectively – so I was generally on my own with Gran.

We would walk slowly along the beachside road together, Gran supported by an old wooden walking stick, to Mrs Webb's store to buy the most delicious pies for lunch. Then Gran would take to the sofa for a nap, while I roamed the sandhills and scoured her bookshelves, reading all kinds of books that I probably shouldn't have read. (Gran loved a good bodice-ripper!) When she woke, we would play canasta together.

When I look back, it's the little things I remember of our time together. Her clear joy in my company, and mine in hers. I remember the cosiness of her house. The ritual of afternoon tea, taken by the fire or outside in the garden, depending on the season. The stories she told of her life growing up in England. Looking back, I wish I'd asked her more about that. That's the thing about grandparents. They have so much history to share. So much has changed in their lifetime ... Gran's life began before cars, well before planes, and I remember her sense of wide-eyed wonder when the first people went into space.

Gran was the only grandparent I knew. Her husband died young, during the Second World War. She was a widow for nearly 40 years. Dad's mother died before I was born and his father soon after. So Gran was special.

When I became a parent, I often thought about what sort of grandparent I would like to be if I was lucky enough to have the chance. I would look back and remember those rituals my gran created for me, hoping to re-create similar ones for my own grandchildren. Now, I can confirm that I'm a much better grandparent than I was a parent. It's easier second time around! As well as having a wealth of childrearing experience to call on, Chris and I are also fortunate to have the luxury of pretty much undivided time to devote to our grandchildren. We're lucky to have lots of contact with them while we're still young enough to be actively involved. We can generally care for them whenever needed. At the time of writing, we're fresh from a seven-week stint with Sadie, Hudson and Murphy while their parents were away on film shoots. Exhausting (there's a reason you don't have children in your seventies!) but at the same time enormously rewarding. It's a wonderful opportunity to really get to know them.

Grandfriends

Of course, becoming a grandparent is by no means a given. There are many of us out there who, for one reason or another, do not have grandchildren in our lives. You may not have had children of your own, or your children may have decided not to have kids. They may have tried to have kids, and it hasn't worked for them. You may be divorced and estranged from family.

Alternatively, you may have grandchildren, but they live overseas or in another part of the country, so you only see them in person occasionally. The majority of the contact you have with them may be seeing their faces on a screen. It's tough if your family are not around, especially as you don't exactly get to choose where they live. My parents and in-laws weren't around when we were raising our children, and it was our fault. Chris and I moved away for work. We never gave it a second thought. The job opportunity was there, so we took it. Now that I have my own grandchildren, I realise how devastating that must have been for our parents, particularly our mums, whose lives revolved around family. And of course, it gets complicated if your child shacks up with someone from another part of the country or the world. Then, even if they do have children, one set of grandparents is always going to have to settle for those FaceTime calls and holiday visits – unless they themselves move.

For some people, learning they will never be a grandparent is devastating. Many simply expect that their turn will come – like I did, they look forward to it and wonder what sort of a grandparent they will be – so discovering that dream will never come true can be a source of enormous grief. It can also be difficult to talk about, especially if you feel as though every single one of your friends has grandchildren coming out their ears. And I'm well aware that those of us with grandchildren can go on and on about them, which just increases the pain.

It's absolutely normal to feel sad. Try not to bottle it up. A lot of people feel their grief over not having grandchildren doesn't 'count' as much as the grief of parents who can't conceive, or people who are going through life traumas like terminal illness, divorce or redundancy. The grief is real. It's important to acknowledge it and talk about it with someone, be it a partner or friend. If your children don't want children of their own, try to understand and accept their choice.

Even if you find yourself without grandkids, you don't have to miss out. There are a number of things you can do to alleviate that sense of loss or grief. You could volunteer in your local school as a teacher aide, or help out with a community group for children. And you can always offer to help babysit your friends' grandchildren! Another thing you might consider is 'adopting' some grandchildren.

As so many young Brits do, Jo Hayes first came to New Zealand on her OE. She always planned to go home when she was ready to settle down and raise a family, but life had other plans for her. Love intervened, and she ended up marrying a Kiwi. The pair had two children. Soon after her second child was born, her marriage broke up, and Jo found herself on her own. One morning, when she was dropping her daughter at daycare, she met an older woman who was there dropping off her granddaughter. The pair struck up a friendship.

'I was feeling particularly vulnerable at the time,' Jo recalls, 'and I said to my friend, "I wish I had someone I could call on to be my back-up." "I can do that!" came the reply. And that's how the first grandfriend came to be!'

Jo thought others might be in the same situation, so she put a post on her community Facebook page, saying she was thinking of setting up a group to connect older people with young families. The post was flooded with comments from people wanting to be involved and asking how they could join.

From there, Jo established GrandFriends (originally called Surrogate Grandparents), a nationwide organisation that pairs older people with young families who have no older relatives in their lives. Their relatives may have passed on, or they may live elsewhere in the country or the world. It is a wonderful way to encourage intergenerational relationships. A win–win.

Jo and her original grandfriend, now known to both Jo and her kids as Granny Susan, are part of each other's families. Granny Susan's own daughter has three children and lives close by. 'The whole extended family has kind of merged into one, and the children treat each other like cousins,' Jo says. 'Granny Susan calls me her angel.' Yet Jo feels it's truly the other way round. 'I don't know what I'd do without her.'

Of course, it can take a long time to find a friendship that deep. It's not always easy to connect with people, and many of us are looking for a bit of help. Since GrandFriends was established in 2017, more than 500 families have joined up. You can apply online at grandfriends.nz. All potential GrandFriends undergo a police check, and families are asked for a history of criminal convictions – this process takes around six weeks. Then, families are connected by regional coordinators. Jo advises taking it slowly. 'Don't rush in. Think about it as entering a long-term relationship. It's all about communication.'

You'll find some hearty endorsements on the GrandFriends website. Here is just one example, from Helen and Peter in Karori: 'We love our wee family to bits … We see them every two to three weeks, and appreciate them including us in so many activities. We always learn more and get to love them more and more. So grateful for all you do. May you continue to have encouragement.'

It's important to emphasise that GrandFriends is not a babysitting service. The focus is on establishing a relationship that is mutually beneficial. Providing a sense of purpose and a connection with young people for older men and women, and a wonderful source of support and knowledge for young families. As the GrandFriends website says, 'It takes a village to raise a family. GrandFriends is about bringing the village together.'

The joys of grandparenting (or grandfriending!)

I treasure those moments when the little ones burst through the door like puppies, full of the joys of life, always thrilled to see me. The special hugs, the quiet moments snuggling on my lap while we read the same story over and over. The trusting little hand clasped in mine as we head out into the world. The shambles in the kitchen when we bake together – yes, that, too! The older ones – the Double Digits, we call them – are naturally beginning to feel the pull towards their peers, which means we grandparents may have to take a back seat for a time, but I know we'll always be close. We've started chatting with the older ones on WhatsApp – nothing like beating them at their own game!

I remember those special moments with Gran. Her specialty was butterfly cakes, those tiny sponge cupcakes with the tops sliced off and halved to create butterfly wings, pinned in place with copious quantities of jam and cream. 'A messy cook's a good cook,' Gran would say benignly, as I proceeded to smear flour and eggs from one end of the kitchen to the other.

I, too, have a few grandparenting rituals. Afternoon tea is one. There's a lot of chat to be had over crumpets and hot Milo. A good, long soak in a bath before bed, preferably with bubbles, is another. Stories I once read to their parents, such as *Peepo!* and *The Jolly Postman*, as well as new favourites, *Stickman* and *The Pirate Cruncher*. We spend hours making playdough 'dinners' and crazy animals. (Snails and rabbits are my forte.) We mess about with poster paint. It's all about having fun at home and slowing down.

We all love jigsaw puzzles. Even Chris, who professes to have a healthy disdain for them, has occasionally succumbed. And, of late, we've been playing lots of card games. The traditional Happy Families is a favourite, as are Uno, Three Up Three Down, Speed, Snap and Memory. We also play board games – simple ones like Snakes and Ladders for the littlies, and Monopoly, Battleship and Scrabble with the older ones. It can get highly competitive, and yes, there are arguments – but it's a great way to learn about taking turns, being tolerant, and being a good loser and a gracious winner!

The beauty of games is that cellphones are not allowed. Not for adults and not for children. A cellphone-free zone encourages chat. We talk about our lives, triumphs, disappointments, fears. Bullying and how to deal with it, the rollercoaster intensity of friendships, favourite teachers, not-so-favourite teachers, battles with parents, battles with peers, battles with us. It's all up for discussion. Chris and I both want to be a safe ear and a trustworthy confidante, and hopefully to offer wise counsel. As 87-year-old Frances says, 'You have a very close bond with your grandchildren. You never lose it.'

Grandparents also have the time to help with the dreaded homework, and it's actually fun! Chris has been a great maths tutor, and I'm not too bad at English. Again, it's so rewarding to be part of the kids' progress, not to mention the fact that it's helped keep our brains ticking over. Many's the occasion we've practised our times tables on a drive somewhere!

The relationship a grandparent has with their grandchildren is symbiotic: they keep you young at heart, while you can share a lifetime's worth of wisdom in bite-sized chunks. Grandparents are naturally a repository of family history. We can tell the stories handed down through generations. Māori and Pasifika elders are particularly good at this, and are traditionally respected by the younger generation for the knowledge they hold. Both cultures encourage relationships between the generations in an interdependent way. The older generation passing knowledge and tikanga to the younger, and the younger helping to care for their elders at the same time as learning the importance of respect and thoughtfulness.

These days, however, the elderly in all cultures are often dismissed as 'not knowing' or 'not understanding', but we actually do 'know' and 'understand'. We have been through many of life's challenges and have come out the other side. Some of us have experienced wars, depressions, stock-market crashes, housing booms and busts, inflationary times, relationship issues, good and bad of all kinds. We 'know'.

In Pasifika families, family includes your extended family, which is usually large. Aunts and uncles help out with nieces and nephews. Elders are responsible for making sure the right decisions are made. They're leaders of physical and spiritual well-being, holders of genealogical knowledge, and navigational and fishing skills. And often it's older women who pass on the cultural and language knowledge. 'I'm teaching my grandchildren that there is a place I call home,' one Cook Island grandmother told me. 'I'm teaching them about island life and culture, music and drumming, and they're keen to learn. I never force them. If they don't want to know, it's sad for me, but as long as they're happy.'

The young are expected to show respect to their elders. 'In the islands, when the elder calls you, you've got to go,' geriatrician Xaviour Walker tells me. 'You don't answer back. Elders are always the first to be served a meal, the first to eat. It's about respect.' However, elders are noticing a subtle shift taking place, where – as a consequence of their youth becoming Westernised here in New Zealand – respect is no longer always automatically given. There can be an element of 'West is best', and that's a cause of sadness for many elders.

Ko te maumahara kore ki ngāwhakapapa o ōu mātua
tīpuna, e rite ana ki te pūkaki awa kāore ōna hikuawa,
ki te rākau rānei kāore ōna pakiaka.

To forget one's ancestors is to be a brook without a source,
a tree without its roots. —Te Wharehuia Milroy

That whakataukī comes from Dr Hinemoa Elder's beautiful book *Aroha*, and it contains wisdom for all of us. Gordon, who I mentioned in the previous chapter, is finding his own way to share his family's history by writing it all down. This way, he hopes to ensure that precious knowledge is passed on to future generations.

Family photo albums are taonga or treasures. They prompt the memories to flow. Our children and grandchildren love them, as do we. Getting those drawers full of old photos into albums and creating new ones from all the photos on our phones and cameras is one of the big jobs I've had in mind for a while now. I keep intending to put those quiet rainy days during winter to use, but somehow it still hasn't quite happened. But, as I write this, I find myself newly committed to dealing with them!

Changing times

Becoming a grandparent subtly changes your relationship with your own children. As adults, before having their own children, they are usually off exploring the world and building careers. They don't need you as they once did – hence that 'empty nest' syndrome! But when they do have children of their own, they often look to you for reassurance and advice. 'Should I take the baby to the doctor?' 'Can I let my daughter go to the mall with her friends?' 'My son is in trouble for being an idiot at school! How should I respond?'

What those of us who are lucky enough to have reached older age know is that, in most cases, 'this, too, shall pass'. When your children are struggling through the inevitable crises of childrearing, that can be one of the most reassuring things to hear. This support role can often be a tricky one to navigate. Of course parenting ideas are always evolving, as I discovered with my own mother! She and I were definitely not on the same page with childrearing. While her babies were bottle-fed formula every four hours, mine were breast-fed on demand. I tended to pick my babies up when they cried, and she told me I was 'spoiling' them. You get the picture! Sometimes as a grandparent you do just have to zip it. If your children don't mind their children staying up later in the evening, for instance, then go with the flow. After all, at the end of the day, you're not the parent. Your children probably have very good reasons for operating in the way they do!

Nowadays, neuroscience reassures us that soothing is not spoiling. In fact, the more a child experiences soothing when they are distressed, the more resilient they are likely to become. Children who receive regular soothing learn that life's ups and downs can be survived. They have their emotional needs met, and they learn to trust the world. The brain stem, where the fight-or-flight response originates, is calmed. These children are able to go on and form stable social relationships for themselves. What's more, a calm brain also allows them to concentrate and learn, to understand the feelings and needs of others, even to feel remorse. All those fundamental human skills come from the simple act of nurture, of understanding a child's emotional cues, learning to tell when the child is frightened, cold, hungry, lonely or tired, and responding appropriately.

Neuroscientists will also tell you that relationship is the primary architect of the brain. Specifically, the relationship between a child and their primary caregivers. The child who spends their first 1000 days in a warm and loving family environment is likely to go on to become a caring, capable, contributing member of society. By doing everything you can to support your children when they become parents – by helping them to understand the importance of nurturing and showing love, especially in those first 1000 days – you are also giving your grandchildren the best possible start in life.

One thing grandparents need to understand is that babies and very young children cannot be manipulative. That part of their brain hasn't come 'online' yet. The brain develops from the bottom up and from the back forwards; the final part to come online is the prefrontal cortex, which is where judgement and reasoning skills reside. Very young children are not yet capable of thinking in complex ways. Manipulation is not on their radar. They are not behaving in a particular way because they are being defiant. Take wet pants, for instance: many children are well into their primary-school years before they are able to stay dry for a full 24 hours. The best advice I ever received as a parent was, 'Go easy on the toilet training. It will happen ... eventually!' That kernel of knowledge has held true for me as a grandparent, too. Simply make it as easy as possible to change bed linen, always use a waterproof mattress protector and be patient.

If you're keen to get up to speed with how things are done these days, grandparenting classes are now a thing. Check them out online.

I know Chris and I are more engaged with our grandkids than my parents' generation tended to be. Their philosophy was generally to spoil the grandies rotten, fill them full of sugar and send them home. That or have them sternly seen and not heard! But things have changed a lot since I was a parent, too. We were taught to sleep babies on their sides; now the prevailing medical advice to reduce the risk of cot death is to sleep them on their backs, without anything – not even toys – in the cot.

Smacking is another one. My parents resorted to it in extreme cases, for instance when I'd been caught lying, but it is forbidden now, and rightly so. I was one of those who campaigned to change the law that allowed people to use 'reasonable force' when disciplining children. The thing is, what constitutes reasonable force? For some people it might be an open hand on a bottom; for others it's a piece of four-by-two or a jug cord on any part of the body that can be reached. I'm glad the law has moved on, and I would have hoped we'd be better parents because of it. However, sadly, our child-abuse statistics would suggest otherwise. Changing the law was just one part of dealing with child abuse and neglect. As we now know, there are many, many other factors that contribute to abuse in the home, including inequality, poverty and lack of access to education or support services. It's a complex problem to address, and it's something we need to work on as a society.

As much as possible, it's important to keep things calm when caring for kids. Try not to discuss adult issues around them. Doing so will only unsettle them and make them anxious. When we're anxious or angry or frightened, the cerebral cortex – the part of the brain responsible for higher thought and reasoning – tends to shut down. We retreat into that primal part of the brain, the brain stem, where our fight-or-flight response kicks in. When we're in this zone, we're not able to think straight or have reasoned conversations. That's why it's important to bring the brain to a calm state. Simple things like sharing a warm drink together or some food can often do the trick. So can reading a story or going outside for a bit. Sometimes when children are in this state, they don't want to be hugged or touched. Try to be sensitive to the child's cues, both verbal and non-verbal. Sometimes they'll tell you more with their body language than they yet have words for. It's important to listen.

In times gone by, bad behaviour in the form of tantrums or emotional outbursts was usually met with firm and swift discipline. Now, we know a bit more about what's going on in a child's mind when things go south – and we also understand that, in our response, we may be unwittingly aiding and abetting that so-called bad behaviour. One technique when a child is having a tantrum is to watch their eyes. Are their eyes following you when you're talking? If not, the child is likely to be in a dissociative state, where the logical brain shuts down and goes into fight-or-flight mode. The tantrum may well have been triggered by something completely innocent, like a slammed door or something else seemingly harmless. If a child is in this zone, it's best to wait. Give them some space, and don't worry about trying to talk to them until they've calmed down and their eyes can engage with you again.

On a lighter note, another huge change is the sheer number of choices kids today have. There's technology, of course, but there's also all the stuff – the toys and clothes and books and everything else that was so expensive back in our day but is now so much cheaper and more easily accessible. If you have the means (and especially if you didn't back when you were a parent yourself), it can be tempting to shower your little darlings with everything and anything that will make them happy! But I would offer a word of caution here: think about the things that you remember from your childhood. Chances are, it's the experiences you had with your grandparents, not the 'things' they gave you, that you most recall. Time is truly the greatest gift of all.

All this is to say, it can be a tough old world out there for a grandparent. So, how should a modern grandparent operate?

Tips and tricks

What children want is love, security, stability and routine. They crave knowing their boundaries and limits. They will begin to thrive if they have those things. Bearing this in mind, there are a few tips and tricks I've discovered in my time so far as a grandparent that you might find helpful, too.

One of the biggest conundrums many grandparents these days face is how to deal with all that choice. Giving kids choices is about giving them some control over what they're doing. The experts will also tell you it's all about developing creative thinkers and future problem-solvers. The key thing here is to make sure the options you give them are acceptable to you! Two of my youngest grandkids, Murphy (five) and Billie (seven), are very particular about what they wear. I am not allowed to choose. If I do, it could well end in tears. Getting dressed can take some time, which can be frustrating in the extreme, especially when you're already running late! I've found narrowing it down to two options is enough of a 'choice' for them. 'Which T-shirt would you like to wear?' I'll say, holding up two. 'The green one, or the red one?' (Admittedly, I usually still have to endure the 'eeny, meeny, miny, moe' thing!)

Young kids have energy to burn, so try to give them lots of opportunities to play outside. Take them somewhere they'll have space to move around, dance, crawl, climb, run and just generally be free. My grandies love going barefoot – just one of the glories of growing up in New Zealand.

Screen-time can be an enormous source of contention. Whether you like it or not, social media is a big part of everyone's lives now. When it comes to our young people, social media is how they socialise. The older ones catch up with their friends online after school, and share their innermost thoughts and homework woes. Banning it outright is a big deal – and, for the sake of your relationship with your grandchildren, probably best avoided. Instead, set limits that follow what they do at home, or that you've negotiated with them. Build technology use into their day, so they can look forward to it. Make it something they earn. Just make sure they understand that mealtimes and bedtimes are device-free zones. (This should apply to grandparents, too!)

A good sleep routine is key to good behaviour. That and a good breakfast! Find out what your grandchildren's sleep routine is at home, and replicate it at your place if you're caring for them. If there's no routine, set one for your place! Kids are just like adults in that way; they, too, need good sleep hygiene. And they particularly need downtime from screens before they go to sleep.

It also helps not to rark them up before bed. (I've found this can be a problem with over-exuberant grandfathers. Chris, aka Poppa, is the fun guy in our house ... but he often needs a little reining in at bedtime!) Sing the songs they sing at home. 'The Skye Boat Song' is a favourite in our family, as is 'The Gypsy Rover'.

One of our special bedtime rituals is a little meditation I do with the kids if they're having trouble drifting off to sleep. I get them to breathe in deeply through their nose and sigh out through their mouth several times. 'Feel your body sinking heavily into the mattress ...' I say, then we start the meditation.

I take them to a meadow in their imaginations, gently describing the warm, soft grass, the scent of lavender drifting on the breeze, the sound of crystal-clear water trickling over the little rounded pebbles in the stream, all in my very best softest, most boring, sleep-inducing tones … How elaborate it gets depends entirely on how tired I am and how tired they are! I always finish with, 'You are safe and happy and much loved, and all is well with the world.' It seems to calm them and usually sends them happily off to sleep. Although sometimes I feel as though I'll drop off before they do!

There are a few things I've found it's best to avoid as a grandparent:

- **Don't try to raise grandchildren like you did your own children.** Times change – your ideas about parenting may not match your children's!
- Don't fill them full of sugary treats.
- **Be strict with car seats and seatbelts.** Follow the latest guidelines and regulations. (Admittedly, this can be tricky when you're dealing with a mid-tantrum two-year-old who's gone rigid and refuses to get into their car seat! This happened to me a lot as a parent, and I found walking away, while still in eyeshot, and leaving them to it for a bit helped. Just a rider here to obviously make sure they're safe before you walk away … and don't go far!)
- **Respect their parents' instructions about discipline.**
- **Try not to reward bad behaviour.** Ride out tantrums. Don't give in!

- **Limit screen-time.** Don't just let them watch telly or play on the tablet ad infinitum so you can have a quiet life.
- **Keep your naming advice to yourself.**
- **Avoid inter-grandparent rivalry.**

On the other hand, there are plenty of ways you can be a fabulous grandparent! Here's a list of top-ten things to try to remember:

1. **Ask rather than answer.**
2. **Be silly and have fun.**
3. **Be mellow when it comes to mess.**
4. **Do things with your grandchildren; don't just give things.** Create experiences you can share.
5. **Avoid playing favourites.**
6. **Take the lead.**
7. **Be a trusted confidante.** Your grandkids should feel confident that you won't pass secrets on.
8. **Store and share family history.**
9. **Keep in touch.** Be proactive about calling and texting. Don't wait for them (or their parents!) to call you.
10. **Above all, love them unconditionally and without judgement.**

Raising grandkids

More and more, grandparents are finding themselves in the position of having to raise their grandchildren on their own. This is an enormous responsibility, especially at a time when you may have started thinking about finally having time to yourself. Suddenly, you're back at square one, possibly raising babies or toddlers, some of whom may have major behavioural issues.

Grandparents Raising Grandchildren (GRG) is an organisation that supports the thousands of families in this very situation. It began in 1999 when a Birkenhead grandmother, Diane Vivian, put an ad in the paper saying, 'Is there anyone else like me out there who's struggling?' A hundred people answered the ad. Now, in 2022, there are 6000 member families on the books, collectively caring for 16,000 grandchildren. I suspect that might be the tip of the iceberg.

GRG focuses solely on grandparents who are full-time caregivers to their grandchildren. They're carrying a heavy load. It's a whole different dynamic to fostering because of the family ties involved. The grandparents may also be having to balance their time between caring for other grandchildren in the wider family. It's tricky to achieve balance when one family needs more help than another!

According to Kate Bundle, CEO of GRG, there is often a honeymoon period when a grandchild first comes to live with their grandparents. Things seem to go along really well, the child is happy to be safe – but once things have settled down and the child feels secure, things can begin to unravel and behaviour goes downhill. The thing, she says, is to choose your battles wisely. 'Easier said than done!' I hear you say.

Complicating things is the fact that there are usually pretty tragic reasons behind why kids end up being raised by their grandparents. Tess Gould-Thorpe, the coordinator for GRG in East Auckland, told me about a woman in her group who got a knock on the door from Oranga Tamariki/the Ministry for Children out of the blue one day when she was in her sixties. 'Do you have a son?' they asked. 'I do,' she replied, 'but I haven't heard from him in three years.' It turned out her son had a partner in jail and three children under three, all of whom were suffering from foetal alcohol spectrum disorder and were on the autism spectrum. This grandmother ended up caring for all three. Her life was turned upside down, but with GRG's help she managed to get through and the youngest child is now 12. In the same GRG group, Tess said, there are also two grandfathers raising their grandchildren single-handedly, and one couple raising eight children, two of whom have autism.

There's a large part of these relationships that rests on loss. The grandparents have lost the pleasure of being someone who can just lavish attention on and spoil their mokopuna. Some are caring for their grandchildren because their own child has died. Others may even have had to take out trespass orders against their own children, which is its own kind of loss. And, of course, the children have lost their parents, and many desperately want to be with them.

Grandparents may find themselves coping with their own grief over the way things have turned out. Most really love their grandchildren and want to maintain that special grandparent relationship, so they also grieve the loss of that relationship now that they must be the 'parent'. They often also discover (as most grandparents do!) that the rules they grew up with don't work anymore, especially things like 'do as I say' and 'don't answer back'. This in turn can lead to grandparents mourning a loss of generational respect – they feel their young ones no longer respect them as elders.

In many cases, the children themselves are sad and traumatised. They may have experienced violence, neglect, drug use or sexual abuse, the effects of which will take consistent love and care, and time to heal. A recent study showed 41 per cent of the children involved in GRG had clinically diagnosed behavioural issues, many of them because of drug use, and some were suffering the effects of foetal alcohol spectrum disorder as a result of their mother drinking alcohol during pregnancy. GRG CEO Kate Bundle says many grandparents are really struggling with behavioural problems. In pre-teens especially, little things can trigger anxiety, aggression and depression. Grandparents worry, too, about their grandchildren taking drugs. To help with those behavioural issues, GRG run caregiver education programmes called SALT (Simply Acquired and Learnt Techniques). These programmes are delivered in a support-group setting.

All children need to know they are loved. If you are raising grandkids, the message is the same as it is when you're simply a grandparent: let them know you love them. In this particular instance, reassure them that their parents love them too, even though they may not be able to look after them. As Gould-Thorpe says, 'The love is there for these children. The child does not have a choice or a voice, so he needs an adult to have that for him, and it needs to be a safe one.' Children need to know they are not the problem. They naturally blame themselves for break-ups and family issues.

'You need to be a stoic,' Gould-Thorpe adds. 'These kids are all wounded in some way, and they can take it out on their grandparents as though it's their fault that they're not with mum and dad.'

GRG is invaluable for these families. Being able to talk about your situation with people who really hear you is so important. It also helps to talk through the bureaucratic hurdles, and learn what you're entitled to. Even if you have perfectly healthy grandchildren, the sheer financial burden of taking care of them is huge. Bundle tells me she's seen many grandparents neglect their own health or hold off on getting their own prescriptions filled so that they can take their grandchildren to the doctor. Furthermore, many families report having trouble finding adequate housing for their suddenly expanded family. Gould-Thorpe says people are often too scared to go to WINZ or Oranga Tamariki for help. They don't want to deal with big government bodies, but that's another instance where GRG can step in. As well as helping to identify income support or financial assistance for things like clothing through WINZ, it can also act as an intermediary with Oranga Tamariki and other agencies. It can also assist you with school and doctor enrolments.

If you are raising your grandchildren full-time, there are a number of financial supports you may be eligible for through WINZ:

- **The Unsupported Child's Benefit** is a weekly payment that helps carers supporting a child or young person whose parents can't care for them because of a family breakdown.
- **The Orphan's Benefit** is a weekly payment that helps carers supporting a child or young person whose parents have died or can't be found, or can't look after them because they have a serious long-term health condition or incapacity.
- **The Extraordinary Care Fund** is a grant of up to $2000 per year per child. You can apply if a child you care for shows promise in a skill or talent, or because they are experiencing difficulties and need extra support. To qualify you need to already be getting the Unsupported Child's Benefit or Orphan's Benefit.
- **Holiday and Birthday Allowance** payments can be used to celebrate important events in a child's life, such as their birthday or Christmas. If your child is on an Unsupported Child's Benefit or Orphan's Benefit, you will automatically receive this.
- **The Establishment Grant** is a one-off payment to carers of someone else's child to help with the costs when a child first comes into their care. This can be used to pay for things like bedding and clothing.
- **The School and Year Start-up Payment** is available at the beginning of each year for each child. It's for people caring for another person's child who need help with preschool or school-related costs at the beginning of the year. You'll have to apply for this one at the start of each year.

There may also be other benefits you are eligible for, so it's best to call WINZ and let them know your situation. You can find their contact details and opening hours on their website (workandincome.govt.nz).

The support that GRG offers to grandparents raising grandkids is so empowering. 'You have to be the squeaky wheel,' Gould-Thorpe says. 'To keep pushing, to get help for your kids.' She's also quick to point out the importance of caring for yourself. 'Remember, you have taken on a huge load, so make sure to prioritise your own time out. Visit a friend, indulge in a hobby, potter in the garden, go for a walk … Whatever works for you that is relaxing and re-energising.'

In 2022, I wrote a story for the *Australian Women's Weekly* about Michelle (not her real name), who was raising eleven of her grandchildren. 'At 56 this is not where I expected to be,' Michelle told me. 'The children are at their most vulnerable stage. They've already had a bad start. What happens now will impact them for the rest of their life.' She described it as a rollercoaster ride. 'It's never always up. It's never always down. It's side steps and down. Whenever I get a call from school, I think, "Oh no, what now?" When things go wrong, we carers always feel it's our fault.'

I take my hat off to those of you who are raising your grandchildren. You are extraordinary human beings. I know you have usually been called on to do so at a time of life when you should have been slowing down, or finally getting a chance to do the things you might have waited a lifetime to do. Some of you have had to give up work, or sell your house, or get a bigger mortgage to move to a home large enough to accommodate your grandchildren. It is, without a doubt, a huge upheaval.

However, please hold this last piece of advice from Gould-Thorpe close: 'Don't feel you're stuck where you are now. Children do grow up, and we relax.'

10

THE R-WORD
Retirement

'Often when you think you're at the end of something,
you're at the beginning of something else.'
—**Fred Rogers, *The World According to Mister Rogers***

At the end of 2022, Gerry Harvey – founder and chair-person of retail giant Harvey Norman, and one of Australia's richest men – told the *New Zealand Herald* that retirement was not on the cards. 'Why would you slow down at 83?' he said. 'It's more interesting like this. Every day I've got all these challenges and triumphs and disasters.'

It wasn't money motivating him to keep going. Far from it. 'At the end of the day, you've got to be happy and healthy,' he said. 'Nothing else matters. If you're useful, you feel as if you're contributing to society, you're building a business, you're doing all sorts of things all the time. If that's your life, then you've got a blessed life. So I've just got to keep remembering how lucky I am.'

My 74-year-old husband recently stopped going to work. 'I was sitting at a computer screen most of the day, and I just came to feel there was so much I wanted to do outside of work,' Chris says. Like me, he's resistant to the R-word. 'Retirement is a category, and I don't like being categorised, no matter what it's called. When I see representations of what it's like to be retired in the media, I think, "That's not a life for me." The ads have lots of shots of happy people sipping coffee in the sun and going off on jaunts … That's not me. Basically, I like to have jobs to do. Maybe I'll never finish them, but I have to have jobs to do.'

My heart sinks when my DIY hero suggests those unfinished jobs might remain so! Have I mentioned I'm basically married to Tim the Tool Man? Chris just loves to build and create things. He's spent 30 years designing and building our bach, and he designed and built an addition to another. No, our bach still isn't finished! It's been a labour of love. He gets enormous satisfaction from it, and he wants that to continue. So, when people ask what he's doing now, he says simply, 'I'm doing my own thing.'

That's the thing about the R-word. If someone asks, 'So what are you doing these days?' and you reply, 'I'm retired,' that's it. End of conversation. Word to the wise: you'd better have something lined up. 'I'm travelling.' 'I'm developing a garden.' 'I'm learning Portuguese.' 'I'm between gigs.'

If anything, stopping work has only made Chris's life richer and more interesting. He's every bit as driven to achieve as he's always been. 'I want to expand my activities and spend more time doing the things I like to do,' he says. 'Things like biking and painting, before I get too decrepit!'

When I ask what he reckons he'll be up to in his nineties, he just grins and says, 'More of the same.'

The right time

Whether you like the word or not, there will definitely come a time when it feels 'right' for you to retire from work.

You will start feeling ready for a change. Your daily commute through rush-hour traffic might wear thin, or you might be over staring at a computer all day. If your job's more physical, your body may be starting to complain about the demands on it. Those daily work challenges that were once so exciting and satisfying may begin to seem 'same old'. You might start to get a sense of déjà vu. You may even find yourself becoming a tad grumpy, dare I say!

Here in New Zealand, retirement is voluntary. Traditionally, once you reached 65, the boss would throw you a party (usually a morning tea with sticky buns), hand you a gold watch (if you were lucky) and show you the door at the end of the day. That arbitrary birthday is no longer relevant. It is illegal in New Zealand to force someone to retire at 65. If work is more fun, you should keep doing it. If you need to keep working due to household finances, you can. Nearly 30 per cent of us are still working after 65, and of those, only a third are doing so because they must for financial reasons. Indeed, gerontologist Dame Peggy Koopman-Boyden thinks even the word 'retirement' may soon fall out of use. '"Retirement" is an outdated word,' she told me. 'Ten years from now we won't be talking about it. Many can't afford to retire.'

Whenever you do it, and on whatever terms, retirement is a transition. For one, it takes some adjustment not having a regular pay packet. 'I sure do miss the money going into my bank account,' 82-year-old Pam, who kept working as a dental nurse well into her seventies, told me, laughing. It's tricky, making the move from a working life with all that it entails – colleagues, water-cooler conversations, status and recognition, a steady income – to a life doing 'your thing'. No surprise, then, that retirement is commonly recognised as one of two particularly dangerous times of life, the other being birth. Anecdotally, we're told that many of us retire only to, within a few years, end up dead. Happily, there is in fact no good evidence that retirement is bad for your physical health!

It's time we redefined this stage of our lives. It is not about withdrawing from society; it's about re-emerging into it. It is not about stopping learning; it's about kickstarting it. It is not about life narrowing; it's about life expanding. After all, most of us will have at least another 20 good years ahead of us. Yes, it's about evolving!

Nonetheless, it is still a transition, and therefore something we need to prepare for. Don't just fall into it. Many of us will spend about a third of our lives 'in retirement', and that in itself is a significant psychological challenge. As geriatrician Hamish Jamieson notes, 'People get to 60 and they think life in retirement will be a dream. My mother used to say, "Too much time on your hands makes time for the devil." Beware!'

The Harvard Study of Adult Development has identified four circumstances under which retirement is stressful:

- when it's involuntary and unplanned
- when there is no other means of financial support
- when home is unhappy and work was providing an escape
- when it is precipitated by bad health.

Retirement can be a particularly tricky time for high-achievers. They have lost connection with their friends at work, they miss interacting with people, they crave cognitive stimulation, and they are dealing with the loss of status or respect. Unemployment and retirement, says Jamieson, have similar impacts. 'It's not good for people's well-being to stop entirely at 65. After the first three months of retirement, many people find boredom setting in.'

Men in particular are more susceptible to depression at this stage of life. They may become lonely and isolated in the community, especially if they have not formed firm friendships. If that's the case, it can be the beginning of a slippery slope into health problems.

For women who've held higher-level positions in the workforce, retirement can also be especially difficult. Recent years have seen more and more women bursting through the glass ceiling into senior management roles, only to find that once they stop work they're automatically consigned to 'secretarial' roles in voluntary organisations and that people expect them to be the tea-makers. Yes, those gender stereotypes are still alive and kicking!

Bridging the gap

How then to bridge the gap between full-time work and full-time retirement?

Many people over 65 would be better off if they could continue their routine lifestyle and work at least part of the time so as to have some structure in their lives. According to Jamieson, it can be a staggered transition. You can work less, rather than stopping completely. 'A move to part-time work at that stage is really healthy,' he says, suggesting keeping work such as consulting or volunteering going two or three days a week.

Dame Peggy Koopman-Boyden echoes this sentiment: 'What I advise is a transition into retirement in your early seventies. Or start moving towards volunteering while you're still employed.'

Norris, in his seventies, is a great example: he used to be a bank manager, but now keeps busy helping others with tax returns and general finances. He's also part of a men's shed group, which makes and repairs furniture and other items. Like Norris, it's worth finding something that keeps your mind active and gives you a sense of purpose. As the loneliness research shows, humans are social creatures. If we don't interact with others, we risk a cascade of health issues, from depression and anxiety to heart disease and stroke.

Finding a sense of purpose is key to a happy and fulfilling retirement, as is a glass-half-full approach. In his book *Aging Well*, George Vaillant uses the comparison of two men, both in their mid- to late-seventies, with completely different attitudes. The first told him, 'Until retirement I loved what I was doing and was much bound up in it … The shock of suddenly stopping and having no way to use the skills I had built over the years was and still is very depressing.'

The second said, 'Every day offers a new experience.' At 75, this man claimed that the past few years had been the happiest of his life. 'Perhaps it is not so important to add up what we are "doing" as what we are "being",' he said. 'What I am doing is probably pretty insignificant. I am a subscriber to a wide variety of local and national charities. I help cook meals for a city soup kitchen and I have proctored statewide examinations for third and fifth graders in a local school. I care for my house and yard, walk a good deal and do some swimming.'

As Vaillant pointed out, the second man understood an important truth: 'not being of "considerable value" at 75 can lead to freedom, not boredom'.

Rewarding retirement

Having a sense of purpose is vitally important at this time in your life. Helen, now 81, lived down the road from a rest home, and noticed a common change in her neighbours from the home. To begin with, she would often see new residents walking down to the local shops, but 'within six months they could barely make it to the gate,' she says. 'There was such a rapid decline. You see, everything was done for them. They had no purpose in life. It was a real eye-opener.'

While there are four circumstances that make retirement stressful, the Harvard study has also identified a number of ways to make retirement rewarding:

- **Nurture relationships.** Replace workmates with another social network. Create new relationships as fast as old ones disappear. Keep meeting new people, especially younger people. The importance of social networks cannot be overestimated.

- **Rediscover play.** Figure out how to maintain self-respect while letting go of self-importance. Try playing pool, paddleboarding, riding a bike. As Vaillant so wisely says, 'Retirement should be at least as much fun as fourth grade!' In a similar vein, Sigmund Freud noted, 'As people grow up they cease to play. They seem to give up the yield of pleasure they gain from playing.' We need to retain a sense of fun.

- **Be curious.** Keep interested in a number of things. Explore. Learning new things in later life has a high correlation to psychological well-being.

- **Be creative.** At the age of 89, Mary Fasano was the oldest person to graduate from Harvard, and in her graduation address she said, 'Creativity can turn old into young. It is visceral and comes from the heart.' It doesn't have to be award-winning stuff – play terrible golf, turn out dodgy watercolours – but live life to the full. It's never too late. Monet began his water-lily panels when he was 76. In the Harvard study, the most creative men were twice as likely to be among the 'happy well', while the creative women were four times as likely to be among them. Meanwhile, the least creative were two to four times more likely to be among the 'sad sick'.

It's important to feel empowered about what you *can* do. Try not to dwell on what you can't do. As Vaillant says, 'Play, create, learn new things, and most especially make new friends. Do that, and getting out of bed in the morning will seem a joy.'

The four phases

Those who are experiencing retirement will tell you it's not a smooth ride, and often identify four main phases.

The first is the **vacation phase**. That dream retirement Jamieson was talking about. You wake up when you want, read the paper from end to end, have one coffee and then another. There is no routine to adhere to, no demands. It's relaxing and you have a sense of freedom. This dream time will last for a year or so … and then it begins to lose its lustre. Boredom sets in. Is that all there is? you start to wonder.

Which brings you to the second phase: **'wandering in the wilderness'**. You really begin to feel the loss of a routine, the loss of identity and purpose. You may feel blindsided. You didn't see this coming! If you have a partner, you may find being thrown together with them 24/7 is not working. Do you even like each other anymore? It's certainly a huge adjustment for both of you. Neither of you is used to having to account for where you go or when you eat, and suddenly there's someone else to consider!

About now is when you hit the third phase: **'trial and error'**. You find you need meaning in your life. A reason to get up in the morning. How can you make your life more meaningful? You may consult, you may start a new business or you may – and this is the option the majority have found to be the most satisfying – volunteer for an organisation you are passionate about. Finding that special something is challenging. Never underestimate the knowledge you hold, or the pleasure you will get from making a difference in someone else's life. You may have to try a whole raft of things before you find the thing that's meaningful for you. It may be hospice, or the City Mission, or teaching English to new immigrants. Doing something good for others is a fine and satisfying way of achieving meaning in your own life.

The fourth phase is when **things start looking up again**. You begin to recover the losses you felt in phase two. You've made new friends, found purpose in your life, learnt new skills and really begun to enjoy life again.

Remember that U-curve of happiness? It peaks again around now! Enjoy it.

11

STEMMING THE TIDE
Style

*'The beauty of a woman is seen in her eyes because that is
the doorway to her heart, the place where love resides ...
True beauty in a woman is reflected in her soul.'*
—Audrey Hepburn

The Western world has long had an obsession with youth,
now more than ever. You're deemed 'old' when you hit 50.
Magazines start doing those articles about how to look 'good for
your age'. People ask how long you intend to stay in your job,
and 'What plans do you have for the future?' Television network
executives and their marketing teams (mostly made up of 20- and
30-somethings) begin to cast about for 'fresh faces'.

I think of my own profession. In television news, as in so many
other arenas, it seems OK (even desirable) to be a craggy older
man. A craggy older woman, however? Not so much! Older male

presenters are inevitably paired with women much younger than they are. It's never the other way around.

There are, thankfully, a few notable exceptions. The late Barbara Walters only retired from interviewing at 85, and Diane Sawyer is still delivering special reports and interviewing at 77. Both incisive, empathetic and insightful broadcast journalists … It's not lost on me, however, that in order to stay the course they each had to endure a lot of cosmetic enhancement. If you're a woman in television, it's best to be as 'fresh-faced' as possible!

No one is immune. When it comes to getting older, so many of us start lamenting the way our looks are changing as early as our forties. (Even 20-somethings are using Botox now!) We worry about wrinkles, grey hair, saggy skin. We find all kinds of things that are 'wrong' with our appearance. Things that need to be covered up. For me, while I was still working in television, I remember I suddenly found myself asking cameramen for a big soft-fill light to tone down that harsh studio lighting. This was around the same time that I began searching out the seat that placed me with my back to the sun. Backlighting is so much kinder to wrinkles!

There comes a day, however, when wrinkles should be embraced. I know this might sound like heresy to some, but really, who wants their granny to look like their mother's older inscrutable sister? And there's also the problem of matching the face to the body: saggy knees, crepey thighs, thickening waists, wrinkly necks and flabby arms give the lie to that smooth, tight, expressionless face.

Actor Jamie Lee Curtis is an ardent advocate for not, as she puts it, 'fucking with your face'. As for the term 'anti-ageing'? 'What? What are you talking about?' she told a Scottish journalist in 2021. 'We're all going to fucking age! We're all going to die! Why do you want to look 17 when you're 70? I want to look 70 when I'm 70.'

Clearly she feels strongly on this one! Curtis, now 64, has been candid about nipping and tucking her own face in the past. 'I did plastic surgery. It didn't work. I hated it. It made me feel worse,' she says. And, as she recently explained to Maria Shriver at the Radically Reframing Aging Summit, her main approach these days is simple: she doesn't bother looking in the mirror! 'I'm not denying what I look like. Of course I've seen what I look like. I am trying to live in acceptance. If I look in the mirror, it's harder for me to be in acceptance. I'm more critical. Whereas, if I just don't look, I'm not so worried about it.'

Fellow actor Andie MacDowell, who recently rocked her grey hair at the Cannes Film Festival, reckons women are tired of the idea that they can't get old and be beautiful. 'Men get old and we keep loving them,' the then 63-year-old actor told *The Zoe Report* in 2021. 'I want to be like a man. I want to be beautiful and I don't want to screw with myself to be beautiful.'

Men get to be silver foxes when they get old. Why is it that they're the only ones who, as they age, are deemed to become sexier? It's grossly unfair. As we women age, we just become invisible. 'Silver vixens' has a nice ring to it!

Jane Fonda has also gone grey, at the age of 85. 'I tell you, I'm so happy I let it go grey,' the *Grace and Frankie* star told talk-show host Ellen DeGeneres. 'Enough already with so much time wasted, so much money spent, so many chemicals. I'm through with that.'

When researching this book, one of the inspiring elders I spoke to was Joyce Lowyim. She's a powerhouse of a woman. Always bright and cheery. Full of energy and positivity. She also happens to run the organic greengrocer and health-food shop right below the Pilates studio I go to, so I'm treated to seeing her often. If I had to pick two words to describe Joyce, they would be 'fun' and 'vibrant'. When I asked her what her secret to ageing so gracefully was, she at first attributed it to her Chinese ancestry. 'I have great genetics,' she said, laughing. 'The ancestral code goes deep. I feel it!' But then she also told me about what she calls the 'secret life of Joyce': it involves cultivating happiness (more on that on pages 285–287), plenty of laughter, positive thoughts, meditating, family, care, love and alone time. Graceful ageing, in Joyce's book, brings wisdom, resilience and maturity. 'Age is just a number,' she says (she won't tell me hers!). 'Fill your life with gratitude, thankfulness, love for self, family, friends and life. Embrace it all.'

I reckon ageing gracefully and on your own terms is what we should be aiming for. With that in mind, what follows are some of the tips, tricks and know-how I've found helpful in my pursuit of doing just that. Ageing gracefully, in my book, is about making the best of what you have, mitigating damage and choosing less over more. It's not about having truckloads of cash to throw at yourself. Take what's useful from the following pages, disregard what's not and add some of your own things!

The skin

Oh how I wish I hadn't fried myself in the sun when I was young!

At boarding school, my mates and I would take every opportunity to sneak away to 'the native patch', a pocket of bush adjacent to the school, and bake in the sun, stripping down to our undies and slathering ourselves in coconut oil. We'd often return from these clandestine tanning escapades looking like freshly cooked lobsters. Some of us tanned, others blistered and peeling.

A while ago, I visited a beauty therapist and got to see my face under ultraviolet light. I was shocked. It was a mass of brown spots. You could hardly see the skin. That's what prolonged exposure to the sun does to you.

I grew up in the days before the slip-slop-slap regime became the norm. We just headed out into the sun because it was the 'healthy' thing to do, getting outside in the fresh air. Applying sunblock was haphazard, to say the least. That desirable golden glow might have made me and my boarding-school companions 'feel' healthier, but as cosmetic physician Joanna Romanowska says, 'Every tan is a scar.' It's a look easily achieved with tanning lotions or make-up. Better to avoid the lasting damage, especially since, as Chris and I know all too well from his melanoma scares, sometimes those scars can turn ugly. Really ugly.

Sun exposure takes a huge toll on our skin, causing it to age prematurely. Romanowska worked for a time in Saskatchewan, Canada, and noticed that the women there generally looked ten years younger than their biological age, because for months of the year the sun doesn't shine. She points, too, to the many Asian women who diligently cover up in the sun and consequently belie their true age.

The message here is to protect your skin from the sun.

- **Wear sunblock** (at least SPF30) on your face and neck. Put it on every morning before you leave the house, rain or shine. Carry it with you and remember to reapply during the day.
- **Cover up.** Wear a wide-brimmed hat when you're in the sun. Put a light long-sleeved linen shirt on when you're out walking or in the garden.
- **Wear sunglasses.** There's the added benefit of less squinting!
- **Avoid being out in the sun** in the middle of the day in the height of summer. If you love your gardening or swimming, try to do it earlier in the day or later in the afternoon.

As we age, we pay a price for sun damage sustained in our youth. The skin either thickens and becomes leathery, or it begins to thin and go crepey.

Is there anything we can do to repair the damage? There is some good news. As Romanowska tells me cheerily, 'I don't have to stab anyone [with a needle] to get an improvement in texture!' Topical applications of retinol, vitamin C, vitamin E and vitamin B3 will help, she says. You can buy these in serum form from most beauty therapists and some chemists.

Skincare doesn't have to be expensive. You can buy perfectly good cleansers and moisturisers as well as serums from the supermarket. As well, don't forget the benefits of staying hydrated. Drinking plenty of water will do wonders for your skin (remember Chapter 3?).

As we get older, the skin all over the body naturally changes, no matter how much time we've spent in the sun. Pigmentation, broken capillaries, redness and skin tags ... none of it is desirable! There is, of course, a whole raft of light treatments and laser therapies to tighten and rejuvenate your whole body, IPL (intense pulsed light) and BBL (broadband light) therapies among them. There is also a treatment called SkinTyte, which uses infrared light to heat the skin's collagen and firm up sagging skin (goodbye, crepey arms!). Laser treatments can help with broken capillaries and pigmentation. But you'll need deep pockets for most of these! In the end, it boils down to what you can afford ... and how badly you want to achieve a certain look.

If you suffer from rosacea (redness, often interspersed with tiny raised puss-filled spots), Romanowska recommends high-potency retinol for best long-term results. And the dreaded skin tags that appear from nowhere? Those can be sent packing with liquid nitrogen, either frozen or burnt off under a local anaesthetic.

The face

It's not just the skin on our face that changes as we age. Alas, it's also the shape of our face!

Three-dimensional changes take place. First, there are the bones. The bony orbits around our eyes become more rectangular. We lose bone mass in our jaw and it straightens out, becoming less angular.

The cheekbones become more hollow and the nasal aperture wider. We lose some support from the bones and the face caves in.

And it gets worse. We also lose fat in the face, deep under the skin, adding to that hollow look. The connective tissue weakens. The ligaments that hold the tissue in place lengthen.

So, the inverted triangle of beauty in our youth – wide cheekbones, narrow jawline – becomes the rectangle of ageing, with the narrowing of cheekbones and the widening of the jaw.

The unkindest cut of all is that these changes align with beauty standards for men, giving them that most prized male asset, the 'lantern' jaw – but not for women. We just get jowly and saggy. Dang it!

Cosmetic enhancement

'I want to grow old without facelifts,' Marilyn Monroe once said. 'They take the life out of a face, the character. I want to have the courage to be loyal to the face I've made.'

She had a great point. Who wants to look like a mask devoid of any trace of life lived? On the other hand, when we're relentlessly confronted by images of variously 'enhanced' faces, it can be hard to be loyal to the face we've made. It definitely does take courage. Some of us naturally age well. Others of us start looking 'old' while we're still young.

For women in particular, our looks are a battlefield. We're bombarded with messages about looking 'more youthful', about using 'anti-ageing' or 'anti-wrinkle' creams and potions. We must look as though we've 'made an effort'. We must be 'put-together'.

And, paradoxically, our look should also appear 'effortless'. It's very confusing. It can be difficult to work out what you want to do for yourself. Where on the scale from 'no work at all' to 'all the work' does 'ageing gracefully' fall?

There's no simple answer here. The best I can offer is to encourage you to find what you really want for yourself. Don't do anything because you're succumbing to societal pressure. Most importantly, don't pay any attention to what those multinational cosmetic companies tell you! And remember, those images of gorgeous older women on ads are well and truly airbrushed, as are most of the images you'll find on your social media feeds. They're all titivated with a raft of filters and other image enhancers.

It's hard to cover up a bad face job. If you're considering cosmetic enhancement, choose your practitioner carefully. A doctor will give you optimum advice and may well be cheaper in the long run.

Perhaps you simply want to delay some of the signs of ageing. 'It is absolutely possible to reverse the signs of ageing by cumulatively addressing the tissues, making them healthier, softer, plumper,' says Romanowska. She notes that most of the older people who come to her for cosmetic work want to make sure any treatment will leave them looking natural. Like Monroe, they still want to look like themselves. They're afraid of the 'sausage lips' look, and they don't want a stretched, expressionless face. Most clients, Romanowska says, are keen to avoid surgery. They are simply looking to make the best of what they have.

Around the time I turned 50, when I was still presenting the news, I learnt we were moving to digital cameras, which are high definition. The techos were excited. 'Imagine how clear the picture will be,' they enthused. Great, I thought. High-definition wrinkles! Give me soft lighting and Vaseline on the lens any day.

After years of delivering some pretty concerning stories on a nightly basis, my forehead had become permanently wrinkled and my frown lines were definitely pronounced. I was drawn inexorably towards whatever might soften them. Botox was in its infancy, but I decided to give it a try. People thought I was mad. 'Why would you want to inject botulism toxin anywhere, let alone into your face?'

My main question was how much would be too much. I soon found out. I had some in my forehead to stop my frown and lessen the wrinkles. But one eyebrow took on a life of its own and disappeared off up towards my hairline, while the other stayed put. Oh no! A permanently quizzical Jude appeared on screen that night. It was a look that worked with some stories … but definitely not with others. Ha! Needless to say, I hightailed it back to the clinic to have it fixed ASAP.

That was back in the 1990s. Since then, I've gone for the odd bit of Botox here and there to soften the wrinkles, but I'm not keen on immobilising my face again. My face is how I communicate. It's part of me. And besides, I'm pretty proud of some of those wrinkles!

The moral here, however, is that it's frighteningly easy to overdo cosmetic interventions. *Friends* star Courteney Cox told the *Sunday Star-Times Style* magazine that she went overboard with cosmetic injections without meaning to. The actor, who's now 59, explained that she'd become critical of her appearance and wanted to chase youthfulness to combat the ageing process. 'I chased it for years,' she said, before she suddenly realised, 'Oh shit, I'm actually looking really strange with injections and doing stuff to my face that I would never do now.' She also realised people were talking about the work she'd had done, and that gave her the prod she needed to stop.

Completely aside from aesthetics, there's also the matter of safety. Back when Botox first appeared on the scene, there were all kinds of terrifying stories doing the rounds. But is Botox really dangerous as a cosmetic treatment? Romanowska, who was a GP for two decades, points to the warfarin she used to prescribe to patients to prevent stroke and deep vein thrombosis. Warfarin is a blood thinner; it is also a rat poison. Romanowska says safety lies in finding the right dose. It's difficult to find the right dose of warfarin: people need to take the dose prescribed, then have a blood test, and their GP will adjust the dose if necessary. Similarly with Botox, Romanowska, as a doctor, has absolute control over the amount required. 'It is much safer in my hands,' she says.

So do your homework. Talk to people, and find a reliable practitioner before you go messing with your face! If you don't, your face could well end up looking like a motionless mask.

A crucial aspect of finding the right level of enhancement, if that's what you want, is your own sense of self-worth. Looking 'good' is as much about how you see yourself as it is about how you actually appear. As Romanowska notes, 'I can do an amazing job but still not make a difference if the mental and emotional aspect [of a client] is not good.' Trying to find the right balance is deeply personal. When Romanowska is treating clients, she says her aim is to make them look age-appropriate. 'Chasing youth can look weird,' she says. 'My aim is for no one to be able to tell my client's had treatment. There is no "one size fits all".'

Whatever you choose, I'd suggest the answer to the question 'Why am I doing this?' should be 'Because it makes me feels good'. Not for any other reason – definitely not to please anyone else! Romanowska points to the example of a client who was in her mid-thirties and had been given a voucher for a lip treatment. She had never smoked, but had the deep lines on her upper lip of a smoker, and she felt she looked old. It really bothered her. 'She had filler and Botox in her upper lip, and came back for a repeat treatment six months later, beaming from ear to ear,' Romanowska says. 'She told me what I'd done for her was the best thing that had happened in her entire life. It made her feel better about herself. She lost eight kilograms through diet and exercise. She was motivated to change the way she worked, and now spends more time with her family.'

There may be something in the idea that feeling better about how you look can help you to feel better more generally. Scientists have shown, for instance, that the 'feel- good' hormone dopamine increases in the brain when people smile, even if the smile is induced artificially by holding a pencil or chopstick between the teeth.

'If we immobilise the muscles associated with the frown, then those negative messages associated with the frown of being angry or sad are not going to the brain,' Romanowska says. 'There is a physiological feedback loop that is interrupted.'

When Romanowska saw how happy that client was, she says she felt 'humble that I could impact her life like that, with such a tiny change'. That was when she stopped worrying about the suggestion that people only get cosmetic enhancement because of vanity. 'It's easy for people to judge in a negative way, and to miss the emotional impact of how we look,' she says. 'What I do isn't about ageing. It's about feeling and well-being.'

The real you

Cosmetic treatments and enhancements of the sort just described are far from cheap. So the question is, do you really need them?

At the end of the day, true beauty is all about what lies within. That's not just some glib platitude. In my experience, truly beautiful people are those who are thoughtful, compassionate and joyous people. They can be as wrinkly as all get out, yet they somehow magically make those wrinkles disappear as their inner beauty and vitality shines through.

Professor of political philosophy at Cambridge University Clare Chambers reckons our obsession with the way we look is a serious public health issue. Her book *Intact: A defence of the unmodified body* encourages us to really think about what we're doing to our bodies and why. Be honest, Chambers urges, about your motivations for any sort of enhancement – be it laser hair removal, Botox or body piercings. Beware both of 'trying to fit in', she warns, and of shaming others for their choices. Shaming someone for getting a nose job or Botox, Chambers says, is no different from targeting their body's size or shape.

We're surrounded by unattainable ideals. If we lived in a world where there was no pressure to look a certain way, Chambers suggests, no one would be chasing those ideals. (And our bank balances would also look a lot healthier!) She highlights the 'cage of beauty', whereby 'all women should try to be beautiful, but no woman is ever beautiful enough'.

One idea she discusses is that of 'shametenance' – all those things a person does in secret to change their body, from dyeing grey hair to wearing make-up. Yes, that includes make-up that looks 'natural'. Entire cosmetic empires, she points out, are founded on chasing the 'natural' make-up look. When you're trying to look as though you're not doing anything to maintain the norm, while actually beavering away at yourself in secret, that's shametenance. Why are we doing it? she asks.

The simple answer is because we don't feel like our bodies are good enough – but 'if we're all feeling bad about our bodies,' Chambers says, 'then it's not our bodies that are the problem'. The problem, she argues, is the 'constant and overwhelming pressure to modify our bodies and the pressure to think of our bodies as always and inevitably failing'. She points to the classic case of trying to 'get your body back' after having a baby. 'When women try to get their bodies back, they're usually aiming for the pre-pregnancy body,' Chambers says. Somehow that body becomes the authentic body, the one 'that's done so much less than you have'. But, as she wisely asks, 'How can it be the real you?'

So, what to do, then? First, take a close look at those societal norms, Chambers says. Recognise that they are supported by 'commercial interests and entrenched inequalities'. Then, give yourself permission to allow your body to be good enough, just as it is. 'It's about rejecting social pressure, not rejecting all modification,' Chambers clarifies. 'But it's also about rejecting shametenance, which is very difficult to do.'

Personally, I fall somewhere between the approaches of Romanowska and Chambers. I want it both ways. I want to feel good *and* I want to resist the pressure of society to look a certain way. I want my face to look the same as my body *and* I want both to be as healthy and supple as they can be for my age. I hope to achieve that through a healthy diet and exercise. I may indulge in a bit of shametenance, probably of the natural make-up variety and a spot of Botox to keep the frown lines at bay, purely because it makes me feel good!

Make-up

So, on that note, let's talk about make-up!

Personally, I love the less-is-more approach. There's nothing worse than slapping on the make-up to hide your perceived imperfections only to have it lodge in your creases and slip slowly down your cheeks as the day wears on. It's the painted pony look I'm trying to avoid! My lovely daughter-in-law Maya Bailey happens to be a make-up artist, and she has worked for a long time in film and television. She knows what she's doing, so I've turned to my 'in-house' expert for advice about make-up for us over-60s.

The first thing Maya says we need to do is review our make-up. As noted earlier, the texture and firmness of our skin changes as we get older, and this affects how make-up sits on the face. A product overhaul might be in order, as old favourites may no longer work the way they once did. A basic rule is to avoid heavy formulas or too much powder, as they can become caked and sit in our lines, enhancing the very things we're trying to minimise. With less firmness and more texture on the skin (aka more wrinkles – she's so diplomatic, Maya!), products are more likely to move and smear, or to wear off, so buying the right formula and applying it with good prep and finishing can help.

Maya also advises avoiding high shine or shimmer in face powders, blush and eyeshadows. Good neutrals (browns and greys) work well with your skin and can be really effective in enhancing the face.

Many of us will see more colour coming into our skin as it thins: dark shadows around the eyes or redness, broken capillaries and sun damage. A light application of the right products can easily freshen you up without a lot of hassle.

As we age, it's common for the eyes to sink slightly and for eyebrows and eyelashes to lose their structure and density. Again, make-up can enhance those features and balance out the face.

Following are some of Maya's simple tips for getting the best out of your face:

- **Get the right base.** Find a good hydrating formula with a light texture. Tinted moisturiser, BB cream or a lightweight liquid foundation can add just enough cover and colour to warm you up a little and even out your colouring without masking your face. Remember, less is more!
- **Set your base.** This is a great way to prevent your base from sliding off your face! Go for a light, translucent powder and dust it on lightly with a brush. Alternatively,

you could go for a good matte bronzer. Avoid anything light-reflecting. Brushing the bronzer sparingly over the skin will give you a touch of healthy glow and won't lodge in the wrinkles!

- **Use concealer.** I often have dark inner corners to my eyes – lack of sleep methinks! It's amazing what a difference a dot of concealer makes on those days. Maya recommends looking for one that has a creamy smooth texture – I've found Yves Saint Laurent or Bobbi Brown are good. A small amount can be just enough to lift and brighten. Concealer is also great to dab over any broken capillaries or areas that may be a bit red. Again, set it lightly with powder to help it stay put.

- **Do your brows.** Sadly, with age, eyebrows seem to disappear … and then reappear sprouting from our chins, or out of our ears and noses. Not a pretty sight! Fortunately, the disappearing eyebrow is easily fixed. You don't need to spend lots having them professionally dyed, although a good professional shaping will give you a great template to work from. Filling them in slightly with eyeshadow can be really effective. Just be careful not to go too dark and heavy. A lighter tone of taupe or dark blonde can give you good definition without the heavy drawn-on look. Another tip: brush the colour in lightly upwards from bottom to top, not lengthways along the brow. That way the strokes go the way the hair grows.

- **Keep the eyes simple.** If you load too much colour and product onto the eyes, it is likely to move and bleed.

A good mid-tone neutral is easy to sweep across the lid. Go for a brand with a bit of pigment and staying power. Defining the lash line and framing the eye will help give your eyes more presence, but keep that line soft. I've found a darker shadow applied in the outer corner of the eye, top and bottom, helps to 'wake up' my eyes. It's sometimes hard to get it in the right spot – especially without my specs on! You might have to gently stretch the eye to find the sweet spot. That magnifying make-up mirror is both my best friend and worst enemy.

- **Lash love.** Like our brows, our eyelashes also tend to take a hike as we age, but a light lick of mascara will do the trick and bring your eyes to life. Maya reckons a tube formula is less likely to flake or smudge. Good old Maybelline from the supermarket is a go-to for many make-up professionals I've worked with.

- **Pick your lips.** You can be as bold or as subtle as you like when it comes to lips. For some people, a bit of colour can really perk them up and make them feel fresh. Maya reckons buying a good formula is the key to preventing bleeding. Line the lips with a pencil, then take the pencil over the entire lip to provide a really good base. If you don't want a full lipstick look, but still need a little natural colour, a pencil with a tinted lip balm over the top is easy and effective.

- **Blush.** Again, personal preference prevails here. You may have enough natural colour in your cheeks, but if you feel washed out it's easy to add a good matte blush. (I've always

called it 'instant health'!) Maya recommends keeping it
to the apple of the cheek rather than sweeping it high.
Again, avoid anything with shimmer or reflect, which will
accentuate lines.

So there you have it! Maya's tried-and-true methods for enhancing older faces. One last note, from both of us: this is just a general guide. It is so, so important to celebrate your individual style. If you have never been into make-up and have no desire to slap anything on, then all power to you. Likewise, if you have always loved a strong lip or eye and wear it with pride, then that is to be celebrated. My go-to non-negotiables are a lick of blush (instant health!) and the eyeshadow lining the outer corner of my eyes. I'm rarely seen without them!

Wear what feels right for you, and you will rock it.

The hair

I've had the same hairdresser for at least a decade. It helps that Bindy Robb's beautiful, airy open-plan studio, Biba, is just around the corner from my home. The best thing, though, is that Bindy understands exactly what I need in my seventies in terms of a hairdo: a no-fuss, fresh, youthful up-do.

It was Bindy who talked me into growing my hair out a couple of years ago. I'd always had it short for television, mainly because I didn't want to have to spend ages in make-up getting it blow-dried and styled. Now, though, I work from home and I'm on Zoom a lot, so I want something relaxed, easy care but still hopefully stylish. Bindy's reasoning behind me growing it out was because it's counterintuitive. People expect older women to have short grey hair, but she reckons that's an old-fashioned notion. You absolutely can wear it long if you want to.

Like many women, I spent years sitting in salons having my hair coloured. I always said I'd go grey gracefully … but when those first grey hairs appeared in my mid-twenties, there was no way I was going to let that happen! So, right through until 2019, I sat for upwards of three hours every three weeks or so getting my hair coloured – and getting increasingly impatient, not to mention stressed thinking about the small fortune I was spending!

So, how to go grey gracefully, then? A lot of people used the 2020 Covid lockdowns to start their greying journey, myself included. There were some pretty horrifying skunks out there! When I could get back into the salon, Bindy came to the rescue, gradually lightening the base colour, then foiling to remove the old colour.

There are, says Bindy, several things to remember when you go grey. What worked for the dark-haired you will not work for the grey-haired you.

- **First, you need to understand your skin tone.** Olive skins tend to suit grey hair, she says. 'The contrast can be magical,' she reckons.
- **You also need to give careful consideration to your cut.** If you want to avoid looking suddenly older, she recommends an edgy cut.

- **If you change up your cut and colour, you'll need to freshen up your make-up and fashion, too.** An edgy cut needs edgy style, and changing the way you do your make-up will help to keep things fresh and modern. You may, for instance, want to wear a brighter lipstick. Taking your foundation a shade darker and using an illuminator on your skin can also help to give you that fresh, sun-kissed look, which goes well with grey, Bindy says.
- **A pair of ultra-modern sunglasses will complete the look.** As well as covering a multitude of sins, they also add a real kick to your style!

Bindy is a big fan of collecting images of looks that appeal to you. Hop on Instagram and Pinterest, flick through magazines, check out people you admire. There are some amazing grey-haired models out there to inspire us; Mercy Brewer, Darya Bing and Linda Rodin are wonderful examples.

When it comes to styling, I often go for the messy up-do these days. I played a witch very effectively in one of my granddaughters' videos, and frightened myself when I saw it back – mainly because I hadn't bothered styling it. I haven't worn my hair down much since! There's one plus about getting older: you can go longer between hair washes as your hair tends to be less oily.

Bindy recommends treating your hair in the same way you treat your skin. Remember, dehydration increases as we age and it affects the hair as well. A weekly mask for your hair will put the life back into it. 'Those little rituals become increasingly important as we age,' she says.

I've noticed an awful lot of hair in my hairbrush lately. It's normal to shed hair on the change of seasons: autumn into winter, and spring into summer. But I've noticed a steady thinning over time, which is common as we get older. There are all sorts of causes for hair loss – hormonal changes, surgery, stress, shock or trauma of some sort. The good news is that, generally, hair loss from trauma will grow back. (Mine fell out in handfuls when Chris was diagnosed with melanoma. It took some time, but it has grown back.)

You may be surprised to know that every hair has a tiny muscle attached: the arrector muscles. They're the ones that make the hairs on your arms stand on end when you get goosebumps. You can stimulate those muscles and glands as much as you want by massaging your scalp.

It also turns out my gran was right when she used to say, 'Brush your hair a hundred strokes a night!' Buy a good old-fashioned bristle brush, and give your hair a nightly going-over. Hang your head and brush from the nape of the neck downwards. It will stimulate the blood flow to the scalp. Regular brisk exercise is important, too, for the same reason. As Bindy says, 'It's wrong to look at hair in isolation. It's part of the whole.'

Avoiding too much heat when using a hairdryer, using less shampoo and rinsing your hair in cool water may all help reduce hair loss. If you notice patches of excessive hair loss, you may have alopecia. Alopecia is an autoimmune disease, where your immune system mistakenly attacks the hair follicles. About half of people with mild alopecia will recover within a year, but you may have more than one episode in your lifetime. Alopecia can't be cured, but it can be treated with medication. In severe cases, you may need to have injections under your scalp. Alopecia can be triggered by a number of diseases such as lupus, rheumatoid arthritis or thyroid disease.

Finally, the last word on hair from Bindy: 'Grey needs energy. If you're tired and giving in to life, you're going to look older. Keep that effervescence going!'

Remember that effervescence comes from within.

The clothes

Actor Blake Lively once said, 'The most beautiful thing a person can wear is confidence.' It's so true. If you're confident in your own skin, you can rock anything. But that said, the right clothes can also give you confidence.

I love clothes. They make me feel good. I enjoy fashion, but I have always had a horror of becoming mutton dressed as lamb. Even so, I have made some big mistakes, and quite recently too, when I should have known better! This summer, I bought a pair of frayed shorts. I thought they looked pretty good in the changing room. I'd been on the hunt for the right shorts for ages, and these fitted better than most. My mistake was that I didn't bend over in them! Turns out a shortish pair of shorts with a wider leg shows a whole lot when you bend over – a lot more than I was wanting to show at 70. Whoops! Those were recycled within the family pretty darn quick.

I first met stylist Sonia Greenslade in the 1990s, while I was still working at TVNZ. When you're appearing on television, magazine shoots are a pretty much unavoidable part of the job. You're expected to front up and bare at least part of your soul to the media to promote your show ... Newsreaders are no exception. But that kind of exposure can leave you feeling particularly vulnerable. A magazine cover is a scary thing. It's generally a tight shot and, unlike television, which is here one minute and gone the next, magazines linger on in shops and doctors' surgeries. Comparisons are drawn. Opinions are harsh. You need to look your best. Sonia has a gift for achieving that. I found her advice invaluable.

Fashion and style are two different things, says Sonia. Don't be a slave to fashion. If frills are everywhere but you don't feel good in frills, don't wear them. By the time you reach your sixties or seventies, you've probably found your own style. You may love boho chic, or you may wear nothing but jeans and T-shirts. Maybe you feel fabulous in a dress. It's not what you wear, but how you wear it that counts. Self-confidence is the key. How you hold yourself in what you're wearing.

Sonia's advice is to be as authentic and true to yourself as you can be. Think of your clothes as an artform to express your individuality and personality. Remember, when you walk into a room, your image speaks before you do. So, have confidence in who you are. Know yourself, and know your body. Also (and this is coming from a professional stylist!), Sonia recommends finding your own personal style yourself – not paying someone to do it for you. The work you put in will pay off. And above all dress for yourself, to make *you* happy, not someone else.

That all sounds fine and dandy, but how do you actually go about finding your personal style if you haven't already? Sonia recommends making three mood boards: one for clothes, one for shoes and another for accessories. Harvest images from magazines, the internet, Pinterest and so on. 'Don't worry if at first it looks as though you're a magpie who loves everything,' Sonia says. 'Eventually a trend emerges. You'll notice patterns, styles, colours.'

If, for instance, you love sportswear but equally love frills, the key is to combine the two in a balanced way to suit your age, body type and personality. Wear a frilled skirt with a sports top, or a frilled dress with sneakers, or team sporty pants and a T-shirt with high heels. Spend some time playing in your wardrobe. You'll be amazed how you can breathe new life into old pieces just by changing up the combinations.

Here are a few more tips from Sonia.

- **Never let the clothes wear you.** For instance, try to avoid tops where you're constantly adjusting the neckline to avoid bra straps showing or excessive cleavage, or skirts and shorts so short that you keep tugging them down! Don't fall into the trap of following the latest fashion trends, like balloon sleeves or maxi/midi skirts, even when you know it's not 'you'.
- **Don't overthink it.** Keep it simple.
- **If you have doubts, change.**
- **Don't try to be someone you're not.**
- **Play up your best asset** – it could be your back, your legs, your wrists or your ankles.

- **The wrap dress is for everyone.**
- **Don't be afraid to buy a man's shirt.** (I'm always pinching Chris's!)
- **If you are fair-skinned, keep black away from the face.** As we get older, our skin becomes paler. Black can emphasise wrinkles and shadows around the eyes and under the chin.
- **Don't underestimate a scarf.** It can elevate a simple black jersey or dress, and can be worn multiple ways.
- **Embrace colour!** Stick to those which enhance your skin tone, eyes and hair.
- **Free your neckline!** Show off your collarbone, and wear boat-necks and V-necks.
- **Be careful of trying to dress 'younger'.** It can just make you look older!
- **Choose quality over quantity.** Look for quality fabrics – less nylon, more wool. Also look for things that are well cut and put together, with no fraying seams or bubbles on the shoulders.
- **Avoid the temptation to wear all your jewellery at once.** You don't want to come across like an overdone Christmas tree!

Dress for your figure

Your height is also a factor when it comes to how you dress. If you're on the short side, Sonia says it's best to steer clear of belts (they cut you in half) and ankle straps on shoes . Instead, embrace those high heels and know that a monochrome palette will give the illusion of height. If you're taller, Sonia says you'll be able to pull off those voluminous tops with slender bottoms.

Sonia also has some specific advice for dressing to your figure. If your waist measurements are about the same as your hip or bust, and your shoulders and hips are about the same width, you have what's sometimes called an **androgynous figure**. Sonia says:

- You can accentuate your waist by tying a shirt round it or wearing a peplum top.
- Go for volume on top or bottom, but not both. For instance, wear a fitted top with a breezy, flowing pant or skirt. Wear a voluminous top with slender, fitted pants.
- Scoop and round necks are good for you.
- Pea coats, duster coats and bomber jackets will also work well for your figure.

If you have relatively narrow hips compared to your shoulders and bust, you have what's known as an **apple figure**. Sonia says:

- Aim for an A-line silhouette. Buy jackets or shirts that are slightly cut in at the waist. Go for pencil skirts and looser tops.
- V-necks are great for you.
- When it comes to jackets, you want ones that hit the upper thigh. For a coat, an A-line cut with no belt.

If your hips and bust are pretty much the same width, and you have a well-defined waist that's narrower than both, you have an **hourglass figure**. Sonia says:

- Wrap tops are good for you.
- Form-fitting jersey knits are also a winner.
- Go for V-necks and round necks, and elbow-length sleeves.

If your shoulders and bust are narrower than your hips, you've got a **pear figure**. Chances are you've got a fairly defined waist, which slopes out towards your hips. Sonia says:

- Place more interest in the shoulder area. On top, wear boat-necks, prints and colours. Go for darker tones on the bottom.
- High-waisted jeans are your best friend.
- Avoid jackets with unstructured shoulders.

I'm a definite pear, and I have to say a pair of Levi's high-rise skinny jeans always work well for me! I also have an orange, blue and pink floral maxidress designed by Kate Sylvester, and it makes me feel good whenever I wear it. It's uplifting, cut simply and well, and it flows when I walk. It might have cost more than other dresses, but I'd rather have one really great dress than five cheaper but ordinary ones. I can slip it on and forget about it … The perfect thing!

Kate's fashion advice is similar to Sonia's. Wear whatever makes you feel good. Play dress-ups. Decide what you want out of the day and dress to suit – wear the floral dress if you want to feel uplifted, the suit if you want to feel powerful, the jeans if you're just relaxing. She also recommends rediscovering those 'old friends' in your wardrobe.

You don't have to spend an arm and a leg when it comes to fashion. There are great bargains to be found in recycle boutiques. It just takes time to rummage through! I recommend going with someone who is a recycle regular. My god-daughter Mattie rarely shops anywhere else, and she always looks amazing.

Once upon a time, I made my own clothes. Then my old sewing machine blew up, never to be replaced. Back then, I held pretty much to the fashion of the day. It was the 1970s, so think wild and bright multicolour-plaid wide-legged trousers. (Hmmm, inspired by Crunchy the Clown, maybe? I thought they were fab at the time! And I could well have been way ahead of my time, given current trends.) One fave was a blue-and-orange wool plaid suit I made at school. I managed the A-line mini skirt, but I had to get a mate to help with the jacket. I did her Latin homework in return, and I remember thinking I had the better part of the deal. Poor Mary struggled for hours to get the orange lines to match up on the seams! These days I'm more confident about what suits me, but I think my sense of style is still evolving. And there are certainly days when I look in the wardrobe and am stumped about what to wear. As with make-up, I'm a fan of the less-is-more approach. Simple is good for me. I don't want to have to think about it too much.

Feeling good in your clothes can give you a definite psychological boost. I know it made a big difference to me in my work. Not the most confident of people, I found that a great outfit gave me a huge lift. I thought of it a bit like a uniform, a shield against the world: wearing great jackets with sharp shoulders made me look credible even if at times I felt anything but. If I went on air wearing something that felt wrong, didn't fit well or wasn't the right colour, it definitely affected my performance. I lost focus. You don't want to be thinking about your clothes when you have a job to do. If you feel good in what you're wearing, then you can get on with it.

Remember, just because you're pushing 60, 70 or 80, that doesn't mean you have to relinquish your desire to be stylish. Frumpy is not for us! And if you're unsure about anything, ask your daughter (or someone else's daughter). Daughters are always brutally honest!

1 2

DOLLARS AND SENSE
Finances

'Wealth consists not in having great possessions,
but in having few wants.'
—Epictetus

It can be easy to underestimate your expenses as you age. You might retire and stop getting a paycheck, but things keep costing money, and everyday necessities like groceries only cost more and more all the time. There's also the mortgage or rent, property maintenance, rates, insurances, utilities ... The list goes on and on.

For many of us, it's a huge shock when our pay stops going into our bank accounts. It can feel like the tap's been turned off! Don't get me wrong, at the age of 65, superannuation here in New Zealand will kick in pretty much straightaway, but that's probably not going to cut it on its own. For the 14 per cent of over-65s who have no savings, superannuation is what they're going to have to live on if they want to retire. It's that or keep working.

Your retirement years can actually end up being pretty expensive. While it's a big help if you're no longer paying a mortgage and don't have any other debt, it's often a time of unforeseen costs, many of which come at once. Appliances, as Chris and I are finding, are not made to last. With unprecedented rainfall comes inevitable leaks and the reminder that the roof needs replacing. Oh, and the house needs painting, and you need some expensive dental work ... and so it goes. And, with the housing market going bonkers, many of those who are fortunate enough to be in a position to have savings or equity are considering putting them towards helping the kids into a home. There's a lot to think about.

It's important to know what's going on with your money at any time, but especially so as you age. In the past, women traditionally deferred to their husbands for all financial and legal matters, and that's led to a degree of financial and legal illiteracy among older women. Thankfully, this is less common than it once was. My generation came along pretty much on the cusp of women taking more control over their finances, and we have the feminist movements of the 1960s and '70s to thank for that.

Even so, author and personal finance columnist Mary Holm says women on their own, in particular, tend to be more conservative when it comes to finances, both before and after retirement. They have less in retirement, and this is for a few reasons. When working, their pay tends to be lower than that of men, and they may also have taken time out of the workforce to raise children. They also tend to be more risk-averse in their investing.

Most couples will happily share responsibility for money issues, but it's worth stating the obvious: women should be across all the family finances. It's important to understand where things are at. It's not healthy for the 'man of the house' to solely control the funds. Women's Refuge is full of women whose partners have been controlling with money, who have denied them access to bank accounts and managed funds, and it's often a form of psychological abuse.

Know what's going on with your finances. Money matters.

Superannuation

It is often said superannuation is a social contract, something a country should do to look after its older population.

Retirement income was introduced so people would have some stability and could plan. When it comes to the level of payment for superannuation, that was originally set assuming people would own their own home or be living in a council flat by the age of 65. That is no longer the case for many. Currently, around 40 per cent of retirees don't own their own home, and most of those are women. In just 20 years' time, that figure will have increased to 50 per cent.

Historically, the government provided housing for young families, and councils looked after the older people. In the 1990s, the old system was dismantled. Now, the majority of the accommodation for older renters is provided by the private rental market, and much of that stock is not geared for older people's needs. It's generally not accessible for those who use wheelchairs or Zimmer frames. What's more, renters are twice as likely to suffer health problems like asthma, anxiety and depression. Older renters are more likely to go to a rest home than age in the community. Affordable, accessible rental housing has to be a government priority.

According to Age Concern's former head Stephanie Clare, housing for older people will be a big problem in coming years. Appropriate, healthy, warm, age-friendly housing is going to need to come from somewhere, and long-term tenure is vital. As the Retirement Commission/Te Ara Ahunga Ora notes, 'How a country treats its older citizens is a mark of its own maturity. How a country equips its people to approach their later years with positivity and confidence is another marker. And how a country assists its people in hardship, yet another.'

Then there's the cost of living. As Retirement Commissioner Jane Wrightson explains, 'We assume superannuation will keep pace with inflation, but as wages rise gradually and inflation increases, superannuitants keep falling behind. Equity around super will become an increasing problem.'

All this means we are heading towards a huge superannuation shortfall. There's resentment in some corners about the amount superannuation is costing the country, talk about the elderly 'sucking up' resources. Treasury data shows the government spent $14.5 billion on superannuation in 2021. By comparison, in 2000 it spent $5 billion. If you add welfare payments to last year's sum, it spikes to well over $20 billion. Of course, none of that takes into account what superannuitants contribute to the economy by way of discretionary and other spending, and through countless hours of volunteering and helping their whānau. Many of us also often continue to work and pay taxes well past 65. 'The people who say the country can't afford universal super,' says Wrightson, 'are generally people who are comfortably off. Generally, wealthy, grey-suited males. That view ignores women and Māori and Pasifika.' For 20 per cent of New Zealanders, Wrightson says, 'super is the first time they've had a stable permanent income'.

Many worry that one day superannuation won't be there for them, but it would be political suicide to remove it. Asset-testing may well be introduced, but that would likely only affect the very wealthy – the top ten per cent of earners – and as Wrightson says, if you're lucky enough to be in that position, then you're likely to be fine.

There's sometimes discussion of raising the age of entitlement, but Wrightson's not a fan of that either. 'Possibly means testing could be introduced,' she says, 'or more likely the voluntary option to defer taking super for a number of years.'

So the good news is, it looks like superannuation is here to stay – as it should be.

Working and studying

Many of us intend to carry on working or studying, for one reason or another, after the age of 65. There's no magic line in the sand that says you have to suddenly stop doing anything just because you've hit a certain age. You may want to remain in the workforce, or you may need to. Either way, you are absolutely allowed to keep working and studying.

At the age of 63, Tess (who is now in her eighties) headed off to Manukau Institute of Technology to get a certificate in counselling. 'I was working at IHC in administration, and I found I was spending a lot of time talking to parents,' she says. 'When I first went to Manukau Tech, I thought, "What am I doing here?" I panicked. "I don't understand what the lecturer is talking about." But that soon passed. After all, I told myself, I was there to learn. I eventually got counselling work in schools all over the place.'

Tess only stopped working when her husband became ill. Those doubts she initially experienced are sadly all too common in older people seeking to continue their education or work. As Massey University's Health, Work and Retirement Study points out, 'There's a strong discourse of intergenerational competition in society that threatens young people and dismisses current and ongoing contributions of the older generation.' This is ageism. You can't get a student loan after 65, yet you are thoroughly capable of getting a degree and, what's more, being productive once you've achieved that degree.

When it comes to the workforce, ageism also means that, for certain roles, older people are completely overlooked. However, research largely shows there is no difference in performance between older and younger employees. Older workers don't necessarily outperform younger. They may, however, be more reliable. Older workers will generally turn up on time, take less sick leave and often come with the added benefit of institutional knowledge which allows them to apply context to a variety of situations.

And yet Age Concern tells us those in the 55–65 age group are finding it hard to get re-employed once they've been made redundant. They do not want to retire, may still be paying a mortgage and need to work, yet no one will hire them. A lot of people plan to find part-time work to augment their superannuation, but that may not be as simple as it sounds either. It's a shock when you're made redundant at 55, then find you can't get another job. As the population ages, this problem will only become more pervasive. As gerontologist Dame Peggy Koopman-Boyden told me, 'We're on the cusp of a new phenomenon as a huge proportion of society is now well into their seventies. However, a lot of employers have never employed someone over 65.'

A common euphemism used when trying to explain away the ageism that operates in the workforce is 'not a good team fit'. As one consultant explained in a study entitled 'Reproducing Gendered Ageism: Interpreting the interactions between mature female job-seekers and employment agency staff', led by Massey University researchers Jocelyn Handy and Doreen Davy, 'Obviously nobody's meant to discriminate based on age but I think people say "team fit", because if they've got a young team then they don't necessarily want an older person.'

This is of particular concern for women as we get older. Handy and Davy have found that, for clerical workers in particular, 'gendered ageism has been shown to operate from relatively early in women's careers'. They recount the story of a former receptionist in her mid-fifties who was applying for a new job. 'On the phone I can sound animated, and I would often get called in for jobs,' the woman told the study. 'And then they would see me and, not that I looked bad, but I looked my age. And they instantly weren't interested. There were so many incidents. They're [places] run by young, upwardly mobile, stunning young women. They wanted a younger person who looked like them.'

One recruitment agency owner had no qualms about stating why he might refuse one candidate over another. 'I think physical presentation is probably the key thing,' he said. 'We place value on experience, but some people have the perception that you're clapped out when you reach a certain mileage on the clock. It seems to be a beauty thing. As you become more mature, some people might perceive that you're not so attractive.'

As another former secretary in her mid-fifties drily put it, 'The best thing older women can do to improve their job prospects is to lose weight, invest in high-heeled shoes and become as glamorous as possible.' Cynical, perhaps. But not far off.

For older women trying to find work, it's demoralising facing constant rejection on the basis of your age and looks. It's tough, and a huge blow to your self-esteem. And as a result, all too often, women are forced into lower-status work like cleaning.

As Massey University's Health, Work and Retirement Study outlines, 'New Zealand has the opportunity to develop the full economic potential of older people by creating flexible workplaces, promoting age-friendly infrastructure, introducing active ageing policies, removing barriers to older worker employment and educating employers about the benefits of retaining older workers.' We know now that diversity in a business is a good thing, and that should include diversity of age.

How much do you need?

It's a curly question, and one that becomes top of mind as the big R looms: how much money do I need if I want to retire?

Superannuation on its own is unlikely to cover everything, so you're going to need some savings. How much? A recent study out of Massey University showed that a retiring couple living in the city, with only superannuation to support them, would need to have saved $809,000 to have a lifestyle with choices. What are 'choices'? Eating out, shopping for non-essential items, road trips, gym and club memberships. Simple stuff. If you live in the provinces, the amount the study suggested a couple would need dropped to $511,000. For a single person, it's $688,000 in the city and $600,000 in the provinces. Even couples living a slimmed-down city existence would need $195,000, the study suggested, and for a no-frills lifestyle in the country, $75,000.

Scary figures, especially if you're already in your sixties and haven't started saving, haven't managed to clear that mortgage, or are still renting and just getting by. But Mary Holm is sanguine about those amounts. She'll tell you there is, in fact, quite a big chunk of people living on superannuation and not much else. It's not ideal, she says, but they manage. The health and social welfare systems will cover them fairly well in emergencies. Forsyth Barr financial advisor Jeff Matthews will similarly remind you that the precise amount needed in retirement varies wildly from person to person, depending on what they deem they 'need'.

And, while it's just great if you already have the savings the Massey study suggested, Holm says those various figures are simply depressing for lots of people. 'They think, "I can't do it and I won't even try,"' she says. She fears a lot of people just give up.

Don't do that. If you feel like finances are way too complicated to deal with, take Holm's words of reassurance. 'It's not that hard,' she says. 'People can get bamboozled by people in the financial world deliberately making it seem harder than it is. You can do it all pretty simply with bank deposits and a KiwiSaver account.'

Here in New Zealand, KiwiSaver/Poua he Oranga is a voluntary savings scheme to help set you up for your retirement. You can make regular contributions from your pay directly to your scheme provider. It's a no-brainer. People should be investing in it from the beginning of their working lives, in order to make the most of the government's free top-up and employer contributions. (The government contribution stops once you turn 65.)

Mary Holm is a great advocate for KiwiSaver. She says it is diversified, closely monitored by the government, and has lower fees than most non-KiwiSaver funds. If by any chance your KiwiSaver provider goes out of business, because the provider doesn't actually hold the money and the Financial Markets Authority/Te Mana Tātai Hokohoko is overseeing the fund, your cash will be moved to another provider. It is worth noting that the government does not guarantee KiwiSaver. And if you are in a middle- or high-risk fund, you will have to endure the rollercoaster ride that is the financial markets.

The next generation will be the first to retire with reasonable cash in KiwiSaver. How do you spend your lump sum? Cash it in and buy a boat? Noooooo! Spend it with care! (See pages 214–217 for more on spending wisely in retirement.) And don't get obsessed with looking at your KiwiSaver balance – once a year is fine.

It's well worth working out a budget for your household. As well as keeping track of the standard bills like power, phone, rates and insurance, it's also a good way of seeing just how much you're spending on the little things like coffee and muffins! It can also be really satisfying to see how much you can cut costs once you realise how much you're spending on incidentals.

Budgeting is not rocket science. Start by adding up how much money's coming into the house. (Don't forget to allow for tax!) Then list what's going out. (Include things like your car rego, warrant and maintenance, as well as any insurances.) Your online banking will have a record of most of your expenditure, but if you're a fan of hard cash transactions you'll need to keep your receipts for a month or two to track those.

The team at moneytalks.co.nz can help you out for free, and sorted.org.nz is also a great budgeting resource.

And if you want to give your savings a bit of a boost, there are a few other options you may be in a position to consider.

Downsizing

There was a clear difference between those Massey figures based on where you live. One way many of us who currently live in cities choose to cut down on expenses in retirement is by moving somewhere smaller.

Holm's advice here is to rent out of town first. Let your home in the city while you're gone. Do it for a year, just to give yourself time to see if it's going to work for you. A lot of people feel they will miss out on seeing their friends, whānau and grandchildren if they have them.

The other thing to think about, as I mentioned earlier, is medical care. What kind of health services are available where you're thinking of going? Is there a hospital? If not, how far away is the nearest one? This is particularly important if you have existing health conditions that need monitoring.

Some years ago, while we were at our bach on the Coromandel, Chris managed to slice his thigh through to the bone while using a Tajima knife. (He was trying to fix a pump connection.) While we waited for the ambulance to arrive, he kept losing blood. It was a very scary time. I was acutely aware of just how remote we were from hospital-level care. When the ambulance finally got there, the paramedics staunched the blood, and I got Chris in the car and drove him 40 minutes to the GP in Whitianga to get stitched up.

While the GP sewed away, he asked us what our plans were for retirement. 'Do you reckon you'll move permanently to the Coromandel?'

We told him we weren't sure yet.

'My suggestion?' he said. 'Keep a foothold in Auckland. I see too many people come down here to retire, only to find in a couple of years that they need more medical care than we can provide locally. And, when that happens, they're forced to return to the city … but find it difficult to replace what they had before.'

Sobering.

Rentals

If you're fortunate enough to be in a position to consider it, investing in rental property might be tempting. But beware, it may not be your best option in retirement.

Jeff Matthews would caution you to steer clear of becoming a landlord in retirement. Of course, he's a fund manager, so he probably would say that! Even so, his reasoning is worth thinking about: the rental income itself isn't usually that high, so you'll be counting on house prices increasing to eventually make a good return. And, as we've seen recently, the housing market isn't as bulletproof as some would have you believe. House prices don't always rise.

There are also all of the same costs associated with a rental property as with your own home – plus a few more. You'll have to pay for maintenance, insurance and rates. There's also the possibility your property ends up damaged, or you could have problems with your tenants. And, as mentioned earlier, the standard of rental stock in the country is often far from acceptable in terms of tenants' health and well-being, but we're already starting to see changes to regulations in that area. So, you may also become liable for upgrading the property to improve insulation, heating and so on. Of course, you could employ a property manager to take care of things for you, but that will erode your profit (unless you simply pass the fee on to the tenant, which I suspect is what most landlords do).

Another issue is that you can't spend the money you have tied up in property. You might be accruing capital on it, but that's only useful once you convert it into real cash – and doing that means selling, which is not exactly instantaneous (or guaranteed).

And then there are constantly changing tax rules on rental properties to consider, which are making it far more difficult to be a landlord than in the past.

Have you gone off the idea yet?

Reverse mortgages

Some people live in extremely valuable houses but don't have much of a life, because they only have a modest income and their house is their only asset. Skimping on that expensive cheese or nice bottle of wine, not taking holidays, not buying new shoes … yet living in a multi-million-dollar home. They are, as the saying goes, 'asset rich and cash poor'.

In this instance, reverse mortgages are sometimes seen as a way to free up cash. A reverse mortgage is where you borrow a sum against the house – typically 15 per cent of the house's value – but don't need to pay it back until the house is sold.

Mary Holm advises caution around reverse mortgages. While they can be a good way to release equity in your home to supplement your income in retirement, she counsels steering clear of them until later down the road. 'I reckon it's much better to spend all your savings and do whatever else you can to provide money for yourself until you're sort of 85 or 90, preferably,' she told RNZ in 2021. 'One exception to that would be people who have got big health problems and saying, "Well, I'm not going to be alive at that stage in my life."'

As Holm explains, releasing some of the equity in your home sounds fine and dandy ... except, in the meantime, the interest on the loan is compounding. 'That's why I don't like seeing people who are relatively young – 60 to 70 – using it. I've heard of people in that sort of age group saying, "This is great, I can borrow money and do all kinds of things." And I think, Be a bit careful. Just be aware what you're getting into, because they're floating rate loans.'

If one mistake people make with reverse mortgages is taking them out too soon, before they've spent their savings, another mistake is not taking them out at all if they're short of cash. Who knows? If you make it to 90, your house may well be in need of a new roof or a paint job ... but your savings won't be what they once were!

The latest, greatest get-rich scheme

Deer farms, kiwifruit orchards, alpacas, forestry, unlisted property syndicates ... There are all kinds of schemes out there seeking investors and promising fabulous returns.

However, beware!

Having given financial advice for 30 years, Jeff Matthews has seen a lot of these schemes go poorly. The problem with some syndicates, he says, is that you lack diversification. The biggest issue is market downturn – in that scenario, some investors may want to withdraw their funds if they're nervous or circumstances change. If too many people want to withdraw their funds, the manager has to freeze the investment to protect all the investors. It may well take several years to exit the investment.

So do your research, get good professional advice, read the fine print and if it looks too risky … it's probably a better idea to step away.

Spend wisely

According to Mary Holm, one of the biggest mistakes many retirees make is not spending enough in early retirement. Now that's good news! This is apparently particularly common in those who grew up in the 1930s and '40s.

Jeff Matthews recalls a client in her seventies who was so concerned about not spending anything that she was scrimping on salmon, which she loved. 'I can't afford it,' she told Matthews. His reply: 'Next time you go to the supermarket, buy the bloody salmon!' She was a child of the Depression, whose parents had had to walk off their farm, so frugality equalled prudence to her. Today, she's 105 and in a rest home. I hope she did buy the salmon, and other little treats throughout the years!

This attitude arises from the basic arithmetic most people do with their retirement savings. Imagine a mortgage-free couple has saved $200,000 for retirement, and they want to spend those savings over 20 years. So, they divide it equally: $10,000 a year. However, when they're in their sixties and seventies, they're probably going to be out and about, doing a lot more – and therefore spending more – than they will be by the time they hit 80. If they scrimp on doing things while they're still relatively young and healthy, they could reach the later years of their retirement with money to spare – and find themselves wishing they'd been less frugal and had more fun.

When people first retire, even those who have managed to pay off their mortgage and accrue some savings are scared of running out of money when they think about how long it has to last them. However, many 85- and 90-year-olds don't even spend all their superannuation.

So, if you do have some retirement savings, learn how to spend them wisely. Plan on living till you're 100. Then break your remaining years into ten-year lots, setting aside chunks of money for those decades. You'll need more in your late sixties and through your seventies than you will in your nineties. By the time you reach 85, your spending needs will be quite small. So front-load those early-retirement years, while you're still fit and healthy. Go travelling, buy an e-bike, discover new restaurants. 'It's about making a relatively simple plan and seeking advice,' says Holm. 'Don't make it joyless!'

Jeff Matthews is a fan of the bucket method. Divide your cash into three 'buckets' of income. One is devoted to emergencies, such as home maintenance or hearing aids or unexpected surgery. Another bucket is for those daily living expenses, such as petrol, food, utilities and so on. The third bucket is for fun purchases – going out to dinner or the movies, a new pair of shoes!

When it comes to getting financial advice, Holm suggests avoiding banks, as they'll just steer you to their products. Instead, she recommends checking out the Sorted website (sorted.org.nz), which provides all sorts of sound financial advice.

Another option is engaging a professional financial advisor like Matthews. If that's the option for you, here's a checklist of things to keep in mind when doing so:

- **Choose an advisor who charges you a fee.** Then their incentive is to help you.
- **Make sure they don't get a commission on any of the investments they're proposing you make**. Ask them to put this in writing.
- **A good advisor will always ask if you have any debt.** If you do, and if the interest rate is higher than your mortgage rate (if you have one), they'll tell you to pay the debt off first, before investing.
- **Find someone you can communicate with easily.** Legal language is often confusing to us mere mortals. Find someone who will explain things in layman's terms so they're easy to understand.
- **Make sure you get them to explain their qualifications for the role.**
- **Find out what checks and balances there are.** Ask, who is supervising the advisor?
- **And finally, make sure they outline how you can complain if there's a problem.**

One final note: Holm gets lots of letters to her financial advice column complaining about the cost of health insurance as you get older. It can be tempting to drop the insurance, if you have it – everyone can do without yet another bill to pay – but as we age, we will generally have greater health needs. There are plenty of stories out there of people having to wait two years for a hip replacement, forced to hobble painfully around the supermarket in the meantime. Holm's advice is, if you can afford it, to keep basic health insurance with surgical cover, but not necessarily coverage for GP visits. That way, your premiums will be lower but you'll have faster access to surgery if you need it.

Helping your kids

One other factor impacting people's spending in retirement is the desire to help their kids.

The traditional way we Kiwis built wealth was by buying a house. But that's not easy anymore. As the Ministry of Social Development/Te Manatū Whakahiato Ora states on its website, 'Demand for housing across New Zealand is growing and more people are experiencing a severe and immediate need. This demand is generated by a shortage of affordable housing driving up house prices and rents. People on low incomes are most affected by rising housing costs.'

This housing crisis has been building for some time, and doesn't look set to go anywhere any time soon. According to a report released by Stats NZ/Tatauranga Aotearoa back in 2020, home-ownership rates have fallen for all age groups since the early 1990s, but especially for those in their twenties and thirties. At the same time, they noted, 'House prices have been rising at a faster rate than wages over the past five years. The Auckland median house sales price in mid-2020 was about 11.5 times the median household income.'

Since then, we've only seen house prices and the cost of living skyrocket further, although house prices at least have taken a breather of late. This may all seem like it should be of little interest if you bought your home decades ago, but it's having a big impact on the parents of those people in their twenties or thirties. Often, the only way the next generation can afford to buy their own home these days is to get help from their parents. The 'Bank of Mum and Dad' is currently the fifth-biggest lender here, after ANZ, ASB, Westpac and BNZ. According to Consumer NZ research conducted over the year 2021/22, parents doled out $22.6 billion in loans. Fourteen per cent of all families were supporting their kids to buy a home, and nearly 60 per cent of them didn't expect to be repaid. They saw their contribution as a gift.

Of course, most older people who have available cash are all too happy to help their children out if they can. However, it's worth noting that one in ten of those families above put themselves under financial strain to help their kids.

Another option when you don't have the cash but you do have a property is to guarantee a home loan for your children. This is becoming increasingly common. Essentially, you become the lender's last resort if the borrower can't pay. Remember, if you guarantee a loan, it means you take on the burden of paying it back if the borrower can't. It's only natural to want to help your children if you possibly can, but be aware your home, car or other assets can be seized if you can't pay in their stead!

Can you afford it? It's a good idea to work through the worst-case scenario before agreeing to become a guarantor. Could you keep making the payments? For example, what might happen if your child separated from their partner, leading to financial difficulties?

It definitely pays to talk to your lawyer and make sure there is a legal agreement. Make sure there is no room for disagreement over whether or not you want the loan paid back. If you're guaranteeing a mortgage, make sure there is a provision in the agreement in the event of a marriage split for you to be paid back, if there is any cash left after the sale of the house.

It's worth noting here that some parents may want to gift money to their children as a kind of 'advance' on their inheritance. After all, no two children have the same financial needs. One might require more help than another. To keep things fair, make sure you keep an accurate account of money gifted to each child. Then you can make arrangements to balance the ledger in your will. For instance, 'Mary had gifts of $200,000 while we were alive. Frank and John had nothing. So Mary will get $200,000 less in inheritance from the will when wealth is divided equally among the children.' This is only a suggestion of how it may work. Of course, you may decide that your children all have different needs and you don't want to distribute equally! (For more on wills, see Chapter 13.)

The big pro of gifting is that your children will have the cash when they really need it. The con is that it may lead to disagreements in the family about who's had what, so make sure you document everything. Keep a separate file for this purpose and be rigorous about it!

And one other thing – keep in mind that you may need cash to pay for your own care if your health suddenly takes a dive.

Further reading

Of course, there's so much more that could be said about managing your money in retirement. There's a reason dinner-party chat often turns to the economy and the housing market!

For now, though, that's probably enough of a general overview. You may want to do a bit more reading. When it comes to money, the more you know, the better placed you are to make the decisions that are right for you.

On pages 302–303 are some of the sources I've found useful.

Above all, don't be afraid to ask for help. Your local Citizens Advice Bureau (cab.org.nz) will be able to point you in the right direction.

DOTTING I'S AND CROSSING T'S
Paperwork

'*A place for everything and everything
in its place. Order is wealth.*'
—**Samuel Smiles, *Thrift***

G etting your affairs in order might not be the most thrilling topic of conversation, but it is an important one. For instance, if you have a partner and they die suddenly, it can be scary to end up on your own and discover you have no idea about your legal and financial position. You may find it embarrassing, but rest assured, there's nothing shameful about asking for help when you need it.

Don't put off dealing with legal matters. Seek advice. Your local Citizens Advice Bureau (cab.org.nz) can help point you in the right direction, or you can arrange to discuss things with a lawyer. There is also now a 'new law' concept taking hold, where young lawyers who are in business for themselves (in other words, not part of a big firm) are offering legal advice at more affordable rates. They're embracing online legal options, so don't be shy about shopping around.

Christchurch barrister Rhonda Powell specialises in trusts, estates and relationship property, and says she's totally in support of people getting legal work done at more reasonable rates. Some legal fees are eye-wateringly high, and access to affordable legal advice needs to be addressed, as it's a huge issue for those who can't afford a lawyer.

Wills

It's relatively easy to set up your own will, but do beware. It's easy to make mistakes. Powell points out that something as simple as stapling a document together then removing a staple could provide a good lawyer with cause to challenge the legality of your will. Tricky!

For estates valued over $15,000, probate is a necessary part of the estate administration process. It involves an application to the High Court for the will to be recognised and approved legally, and it can take time and work. It can be a thorny task, but you can obtain assistance from a lawyer if need be. When it comes to probate, Powell explains, the High Court is particular about the smallest detail. Common mistakes include putting things in the will that shouldn't be there, like trust assets. Specialist advice is needed for succession planning involving trusts.

If you have a pretty simple life and your wishes for disbursement are not complicated, then a will that you draft yourself is OK. You can find templates online. However, it's highly recommended that you get a reputable lawyer to check it once you've made your decisions. That way you can avoid discord and heartbreak in the family later.

Be aware that wills are specific. There's not a lot of wriggle room. For instance, you might put a clause in your will stating, 'I leave my Honda Jazz to Pamela.' But then you sell your Honda and buy a Nissan Leaf instead. If you forget to change your will, Pamela may be left without a set of wheels.

If you want to protect your will, the best thing to do is sit down with your family and talk about your wishes. Explain things to them, and give them the opportunity for feedback. Let them raise any concerns they may have. According to Rhonda Powell, this offers protection on two fronts: it stops them feeling they haven't had an input, and if there are any disagreements later, you or your lawyer can say, 'You were told about this and you chose not to question it.'

There's also the delicate question of how much to tell your children about your finances. Mary Holm is an advocate for being open. It's a common story that some children need more help than others, and it's so much easier if there's goodwill among siblings. For instance, you can explain, 'We're going to leave more to your brother, because his needs are greater than yours.' Being open can avoid problems when you're not there to explain things. Money can do strange things to people's behaviour, especially when they're grieving. And sometimes it's not your children who are the problem, but their partners. One financial advisor interviewed for this book still remembers how mortified a healthy client in her seventies was when she overheard her son's second wife talking about what kind of sports car she was going to get when the client died!

Living wills

A living will, or an advance directive, specifies what you want to happen if you are physically or mentally unable to make your own decisions about the care you want to receive. It allows you to specify whether or not you want to be resuscitated, or when you would prefer to have life support turned off. It can also cover the sort of treatment you would prefer, the drugs you want to avoid, and even where you want to be treated – in a hospital, at home, or in a hospice.

I should say at this point that you must be 'legally competent' to make an advance directive. That means you must be of sound mind and able to make a rational choice.

It's a good idea to talk this through with your GP. Once you've made your decisions and drawn up the document, keep a copy for yourself and give copies to your family or closest friends, so they understand your wishes – this will help avoid a situation where family members disagree over whether to turn off life support. It is worth noting that you can't demand or refuse anything in the document that you couldn't demand or refuse while conscious and competent. Assisted dying is also not available under a living will, as you must be competent to make an informed decision about it in order to be eligible for it.

A living will is definitely on my to-do list – at my age I have a horror of being 'kept alive' and confined to my bed for the rest of my life. You can ask a lawyer to draw one up or do it yourself, but it should be signed, witnessed and dated.

One thing to keep in mind: your health provider will consider various factors before deciding whether they should follow your advance directive, such as if you were mentally competent, were sufficiently informed, and the directive is up to date.

Enduring Power of Attorney

As you get older, you might also consider appointing someone close to you as your Enduring Power of Attorney (POA), so they can make legal decisions on your behalf should you be deemed unable to make them yourself. In our case, Chris and I have opted to appoint our children. One of them has POA over our health and welfare needs, and the other two have POA over our financial matters. Talk through your wishes with your appointees, so they understand exactly what you want to happen. A lawyer will then draw up the documents for you. A court or a qualified health provider will rule about whether or not you are capable of making your own decisions.

In addition, it's a good idea to have a notebook or file on your computer where you note down all your important contacts: your lawyer, accountant, doctor, bank and so on. Include your Inland Revenue Department (IRD) and National Health Index (NHI) numbers, as well as any bank accounts you hold. You might also consider keeping all your passwords in a verified secure password manager app, and letting someone you trust know how to access it, in case you're not able to do so.

New relationships

So, you've finally met the man or woman of your dreams in your retirement years? It might be easier if you decide not to live together! You will both most likely have children of your own, not to mention houses and other trappings that you bring to the relationship. Sometimes it's simpler to keep those things separate.

Pre-nups

Many people in their sixties, seventies and beyond are on their second or third marriages. Pre-nups may be an uncomfortable subject to bring up in the first flush of romance, but they can save a lot of heartache later. Formally known as a Contracting Out Agreement, a pre-nup allows a couple to divvy up the money in the relationship according to different tailor-made rules, if they're not wanting to share their accumulated wealth equally, in the event of a break-up.

When entering into a new relationship, Rhonda Powell recommends that, out of respect for the other person, you discuss all possible scenarios in a realistic way before committing to a financial plan. It might feel a little uncomfortable and calculated in the first instance, but it may avoid an expensive and lengthy dispute later on, if the worst happens and the relationship turns pear-shaped.

Powell says families need to consider three issues:

1. **The pre-nup.** Who gets what if the couple splits?
2. **What about the house?** Find a fair way to either divvy up the proceeds of a sale or compensate the partner who has to move out.
3. **Family trusts.** If trusts are involved, there needs to be succession planning to see how the trust sits in relation to the pre-nup and the house.

Check out MoneyHub (moneyhub.co.nz) for a comprehensive, easy-to-follow guide on pre-nups and how to arrange your own. Just remember, it is a legal document and will need to be witnessed by a lawyer. Both parties should have separate legal advice to make sure it's fair.

Retirement villages

Most villages offer a 'Licence to Occupy' arrangement, which means you buy the licence to occupy your villa or apartment for your lifetime. Then, when you die, the villa licence is sold by the village management, and your estate gets back around two thirds of what you originally paid for your licence. Your estate generally doesn't get any capital gain on the property – that goes to the village. Many people find this arrangement overly greedy on the village's part, but it is, after all, a business. They must make their money somewhere. It's incumbent on villages, in legislation, to be upfront about these costs.

If you decide to move into a village, make sure you understand exactly what will happen when you or your estate need to sell your apartment or villa. As Retirement Commissioner Jane Wrightson noted in an interview with me, 'The normal checks and balances are not as strong as they should be. When moving in, there is no negotiating room in the contracts. People are generally happy while living there, but when they move out or die, the length of time it takes to sell a villa or apartment and the amount of ongoing costs and cost of renovation is debatable.'

Work is underway to address these issues, but do make sure you read the small print! Of course, your lawyer should be across all the paperwork and have answered all your questions before you sign on the dotted line.

Trusts

Trusts used to be a way of protecting your assets from the tax man, because trust funds would be taxed at a lower rate.

A common reason to have a trust these days is to protect your interests should there be a relationship property dispute, especially for people on their second or third marriage or relationship. Here, it's worth noting that, under the *Property (Relationships) Act*, inherited funds are usually not considered relationship property unless used for the 'common purpose and benefit' of the family, or the assets purchased from an inheritance are placed in joint names. For example, if you have bankrolled part of your family home with the inheritance your grandmother left you, then it *is* considered part of relationship property. If you want to avoid this occurring, consult your lawyer before spending inheritance money on joint debts or assets – as it may be possible to contract out of this usual arrangement.

Rhonda Powell sees a lot of New Zealanders treating trust assets as if they're the individual's own assets. They're not. Every decision made by the trust has to be unanimously agreed by all the trustees.

It is generally too late to set up a trust once you have retired. The IRD will look back at the trust over a period of years to check the gifting. They will be able to see if it's a tax-avoidance ploy and will tax you retrospectively. In this instance, trustees may have to use trust assets to repay the debt.

If you are in a business where being sued could be a possibility, then it could be a good idea to have your personal assets in a trust. For instance, if you're a builder and an unhappy client decides to sue, your family home could theoretically be vulnerable. Talk to a lawyer or an accountant for further information.

Beware of scams!

The big, wide, wonderful world of the internet is a happy hunting ground for scammers.

Those of us who are not particularly internet savvy can often be tricked into believing we're doing the right thing when we share personal information online. Scammers often say they're from familiar companies like Spark or One New Zealand, and will often claim there is some technical problem they can only fix by getting remote access to your computer or device.

Don't ever give anyone you don't personally know your computer password. If you give it to a scammer, they will be able to access your internet banking, scans of passports and driver's licences, health information – you name it, they will find a way to get it. They may even install viruses and spyware onto your computer. If you're the slightest bit unsure, don't do it.

Older people are particularly vulnerable to financial abuse, because financial literacy and capacity often decrease with age. What's more, those unscrupulous vipers that make it their business to scam people out of their hard-earned cash know this, and therefore zero in on us. Be wary. It is so tempting to look for better returns on your investment. It's human nature to want to do better, especially if you hear of others reaping rewards from the latest 'sure-fire' investment opportunity.

The Covid pandemic has seen a spike in scams involving perfectly legitimate couriers or carriers. Like everyone else, scammers pivoted during the lockdowns and spotted an opportunity with all the online shopping deliveries being made. I've had a number of emails announcing that a courier company has a delivery for me, and just needs to 'confirm my details'. These emails claim to be from companies I'm familiar with or have used in the past. I so nearly fell for it. Fortunately, I checked the sender's email address, and sure enough it was unintelligible. It was a scam.

If you're ever suspicious about an email, check the sender's address. They may be purporting to come from IRD, but the address may say ird@mrhenterprises.com or something similar – a dead giveaway. Sometimes, they may be a little closer to what you'd expect, merely substituting one or two letters, so pay close attention: if it's from ivan@vadofone.com, it's not your friendly Vodafone assistant! I've used this technique many times when feeling uneasy about an email, and I've always discovered a strange address.

Scammers can also often be detected by faults in their grammar or spelling. If an email is written in very poor English, it is quite likely from a scammer, particularly if they're asking for your login details or passwords.

Email phishing has become increasingly common. This is when scammers use fraudulent emails, again often from familiar companies or organisations, to try to get personal information from people. Church congregations are particularly targeted by phishers.

Remember, legitimate organisations never ask for passwords or banking information outside their secure websites.

In particular, beware of social media scams, such as fake competitions or scams targeting buyers and sellers on online marketplaces. Be careful when you buy tickets for concerts or shows from individuals. We all know people who've turned up at the stadium only to find their ticket is not legitimate. As recommended on the Age Concern website (ageconcern.org.nz), if you do want to buy re-sold tickets, it's best to look at a trusted site like Ticketmaster Resale (www.ticketmaster.co.nz/ticketmaster-resale). Fake online competitions will often ask for your personal details; never give them.

And just when you thought you had the world of fakery well and truly sussed, along come fake invoices. They look just like the real thing, only you've never ordered or received the product or service you're being invoiced for. The invoice will look completely valid, but the bank account details will belong to an individual looking to get rich quick.

And then there are the romance scams: when an impossibly tall, dark, gorgeous stranger tries to form a relationship with you online in an effort to do you out of your savings. The scammer will often use a fake profile made up of photos and information from random people they have found online. This can happen on email, dating websites and social media.

There are three big red flags that you may have given your heart to a scammer:

1. They are moving too fast – hot and heavy and a bit pushy.
2. They have sob stories about problems that they need money to solve.
3. They make a lot of excuses to avoid video-chatting or meeting you in person.

Never send money to anyone you have not met in person or do not know. If you think your new romantic partner may be a scammer, why not run an image check on them? You can search Google using images just as you can search using words, and this will allow you to see if the images they've sent are being used in other places on the internet. Just google 'reverse image search' and you will find details of how to do this.

Age Concern's website has great information about how to stay safe online. Among its tips:

- Be suspicious if you receive a random phone call.
- Shield your PIN whenever using your debit card.
- Never give personal information over the phone.
- Keep your computer updated.
- Use two-factor authentication (this can be your password plus a PIN, a fingerprint or a code sent to your phone or email, among other things).
- Shred documents containing personal information.
- Use reputable online payment systems like PayPal or ApplePay.
- Avoid internet cafes or public hotspots when dealing with personal data.

Age Concern also provides a list of the various organisations which you can report particular scams to.

Finally, there's that horrible elephant in the room: elder financial abuse. I hate to think about someone abusing an older family member's trust, but believe me, it happens all the time. Elder financial abuse is rife. It can start innocently enough: 'I have her PIN, I'll just buy her this ...' It ends with the abuser expecting payouts. And it's much more common than people think. One in ten older New Zealanders experiences some kind of elder abuse.

If this is something that's worrying you, you can call 0800 EA NOT OK (0800 32 668 65) or email support@elderabuse.nz. If you call, you'll be put in touch with a trained coordinator who will work with you to make sure you're safe and to help manage the risk. They will identify other organisations that can help, such as police, lawyers, banks, health professionals and government agencies. You are not alone.

14

NOT BUYING GREEN BANANAS!
Death

'Death is not a battle we have lost. Death is not a failure of will. Death is not something we have let happen. Dying is living.'

—Leslie Blackhall, 'Living, Dying and the Problem with Hope', TEDxTalk

There is nothing surer in this life than that we are all going to die. Yes, dying is part of living – and yet it is so very difficult to have conversations about death and dying. Most of us put it in the too-hard basket. The urge to survive is strong and although death is inevitable, we are, many of us, in denial. Older age is not synonymous with being 'glad to die'.

We all want to die swiftly and painlessly. That's what Leslie Blackhall, the section head for palliative care at UVAHealth in Charlottesville, Virginia, would call 'the off-button theory of death'. The fact is, very few of us will be lucky enough to go that way.

'I'm not afraid of death,' 87-year-old Frances told me. 'I'm afraid of how I'm going to die.'

That's it, isn't it? That's what I'm afraid of, too.

I find New Zealand's recently introduced assisted dying service some comfort. At least I know that, should I find myself experiencing unbearable suffering from a terminal illness, I may be able to make an informed decision to end my own life. I am conflicted when I say this, as I'm also a patron of Harbour Hospice on Auckland's North Shore. As a sector, hospices did not support any change to the legislation around euthanasia or physician-assisted death. In 2015, when this legislation was brought before the Health Select Committee, Hospice New Zealand made a submission outlining their stance. 'Hospice services and palliative care, as defined by the World Health Organisation [sic], "intends neither to hasten or postpone death",' their submission stated. 'This is the cornerstone of hospice care in New Zealand. Euthanasia and physician-assisted death goes against this because it hastens death.'

Many people are unaware of what, exactly, a hospice is. The hospice philosophy is that death is a natural part of life and that, with the right palliative care – meaning to relieve pain, without treating its cause – a person with a life-limiting condition can still have a good quality of life, right till the very end. Hospices aim to provide the very best possible palliative care for the dying, easing the suffering of the terminally ill while helping their loved ones on their journey, too.

I know a lot of people are frightened of turning to a hospice, because they see it as the end of the road. They equate it with the loss of hope. Some people do die in the hospice in patient units, but a hospice stay doesn't necessarily mean you'll never go home. In fact, some patients live longer under hospice care. Hospices aim to balance your medications to alleviate your pain so that you can return home and remain in the care of those who are closest to you, with the support of a hospice nurse, who will visit you there. I have seen many close friends through hospice care. All of them have been enormously grateful for the tender, thoughtful and expert attention they received. Hospices also provide invaluable support to the patient's family though their counselling services.

The reality is, our bodies are not designed to last forever. Old age brings with it inevitable deterioration. We might all want that peaceful, comfortable, dignified death ... but not right now, thanks. We want it later. As a result, there will be numerous interventions along the way that will extend our lives. Most of the time, those interventions are welcome blessings. Sometimes, though, prolonging life may well come at the cost of a person's right to that dignified death we all hope for.

Accepting the end

According to Ken Hillman, a professor of intensive care at the University of New South Wales and author of *A Good Life to the End*, 'Dying in the elderly has been hijacked.'

It's a pretty refreshing admission, especially from someone who researches the pointy end of life. The way he sees it, hospitals' treatment of older patients who are dying is similar to the way women giving birth were treated in the 1950s and '60s. Back then, women gave birth on their backs on a bed, often with their legs in stirrups; the baby was removed and put in a bassinet in a nursery, along with lots of other babies in bassinets; and fathers were not allowed to be part of the process. The whole thing was taken out of the birthing mother's hands. Hillman's view is that the dying have been similarly disenfranchised.

Older patients often ask, 'What is wrong with me?' But, as Hillman says, there is no single diagnosis for old age. It is usually a combination of diseases that add up to something with no name. Hillman prefers to call it 'frailty'. And, despite all our medical advances, age-related frailty, he says, is not curable.

Hillman and his colleague Magnolia Cardona began looking for more accurate ways to identify patients at the end of their life. They acknowledged the pressure on doctors – both as part of their role and from society – to continue using the technology available to them to prolong life, even in futile situations. However, Hillman and Cardona's idea was to involve patients and their families in discussions, so a more appropriate management plan could be put in place.

Eventually, they developed the CriSTAL (Criteria for Screening and Triaging to Appropriate aLternative care) tool, and it has since become the gold standard in Australia, the US and Europe. At its heart is a focus on empowering patients and carers with choices about the patient's treatment. It enables practitioners to identify those patients nearing the end of their lives, to assess their risk of death, and to avoid potentially harmful and unnecessary treatment. Among the criteria included in the assessment are age, deterioration, co-morbidities and cognitive impairment. More appropriate management options could include sedation to minimise pain and distress, spiritual support and home-based palliative care.

The tool is in no way meant to dictate whether or not a patient should receive life-sustaining therapy. Instead, it is designed to help doctors and patients and their families have honest conversations about treatment.

Would patients like to continue aggressive treatment, to be in and out of hospital over weeks, months, possibly years?

Or would they like to receive palliative care that mitigates their most distressing symptoms and allows them to spend the rest of their days at home?

About 70 per cent of people say they'd rather die at home than in hospital. Unfortunately, the reverse is true: about 70 per cent of us die in hospital. Hillman openly admits that doctors find it difficult to recognise when people are at the end of their life. He says doctors need to be more honest about the limitations of modern medicine, and notes, 'I seldom do a ward round with colleagues when one of us doesn't say, "Please don't let this happen to me."'

The long-term solution, he says, is for those who want control over their end of life to sign an advance directive, or living will (see pages 224–225). This will help to ensure you avoid unnecessary and painful interventions. He also notes that doctors in the community should be empowered to manage end-of-life care, and carers should be able to access respite care for their loved ones.

When that happens, Hillman says, a dignified death at home should be possible.

The next great adventure

Fear of death is basically a fear of the unknown. But as Harry Potter's wise old headmaster, Albus Dumbledore, tells him in *Harry Potter and the Philosopher's Stone*, 'To the well-organised mind, death is but the next great adventure.'

When I think about death, I like to think about Steve Jobs's last words. The founder of Apple died of pancreatic cancer at the young age of 56, and his last words, reportedly delivered with such wonder, were, 'Oh wow, oh wow, oh wow!'

What caused that wonder? Was he seeing his life pass before him? Or was it something more?

To be less afraid of death and dying, we need to be able to talk about it more. Easy to say, I know, when it's not on your immediate horizon. But I'm reliably informed by two of my Harry Potter expert grandchildren, Sadie and Hudson, that when Dumbledore referred to the 'well-organised mind', he was talking about a mind that had taken time to prepare itself for death. A mind that had lived life to the full and was ready to launch into the next great adventure. I love that sentiment.

It's not far off something Morrie Schwartz told Mitch Albom: 'Learn how to live and you'll know how to die; learn how to die and you'll know how to live.'

So, what should we do with the time we have left? How do we prepare our minds to be well-organised?

'Be present for the life we actually have,' Leslie Blackhall says. 'What you're doing right now, this is your bucket list! ... If we can accept that dying is part of living, we can live a fuller, richer life right now.'

None of us knows what is in store for us after we die. Let's hope for adventure – and, in the meantime, let's make the most of the days left to us!

As one of the wise people I interviewed for this book told me, 'A sense of humour helps. At our age, you don't ever buy green bananas!'

Funerals and paperwork

My first experience of organising a funeral was for the death of my dad. I hadn't realised embalming was optional. I remember going to see him in his coffin at the funeral home after he'd been embalmed. I wish I hadn't. I wanted to remember him the way he was, complete with all his wonderful, hard-won wrinkles. The waxy, smooth face that confronted me just wasn't him. Of course, sometimes embalming is the best option, especially if close family members are not able to be there immediately after death.

There's a lot about the ins and outs of funerals that many of us only learn on the spot. Forewarned is forearmed when it comes to arranging funerals, and a little advance knowledge of what's involved goes a long way.

Funeral directors can be a wonderful support at this very difficult and emotional time. We relied heavily on ours when Dad died, especially when it came to ensuring all the paperwork was filed. Good funeral directors will generally be happy to have as much or as little involvement as you decide.

If you want to do the paperwork yourself, you can access all the advice you need on the Department of Internal Affairs/Te Tari Taiwhenua website (dia.govt.nz). The law requires that all deaths should be notified to the Registrar of Births, Deaths and Marriages/Whānautanga, Matenga, Mārenatanga within three working days of burial or cremation. You will need to provide a death certificate, and if someone dies as a result of illness you will need a doctor to sign a medical certificate determining the cause of death.

You'll need the following documents from the deceased to help you fill out the forms:

- birth certificate
- passport
- marriage or civil union certificate
- parents' birth and marriage certificates
- military service records.

I even know some very organised people who've already sorted the relative documents to make it easier for their children or partners in the event of their death. It's a great idea. It certainly takes the pressure off those who are struggling with their grief.

There's also the social media tidy-up to deal with. Yes, it's a sign of the times. You can find information about how to remove or deactivate a deceased person's profile in the help sections of most platforms, including Facebook, Instagram and Twitter. There are also a number of online sources to guide you on what to do with a person's social media accounts when they die.

When it comes to arranging the funeral, it may be reassuring to know that it doesn't have to cost more than you can afford. A funeral is about the coming together of family and friends to grieve, remember and support each other. That's what makes it meaningful. Eastern Bay Villages/Te Kokoru Manaakitanga in Whakatāne is an example of one community group looking for low-cost solutions for people who can't afford the cost of a professional funeral director. In particular, they are wanting to rediscover traditional funeral rites. Māori are weaving whāriki, or mats, to use instead of coffins, and coffin-making clubs have put woodworking skills to good use helping others in a time of need.

It's worth noting that neither embalming nor coffins are essential. Depending on personal beliefs or cultural practices, some prepare their loved one for burial themselves, wrapping the body in a shroud. Others opt for a natural burial – a biodegradable coffin is placed in a shallow plot, which is overplanted with natives. There are no markers, and the plants absorb nutrients from the body, growing into a living memorial. It is currently possible to have a natural burial in Auckland, Wellington and Nelson.

Family-led services have become increasingly popular as funerals become more personal and less formal. We recently attended one such service for a farming friend of ours. It was led by family members in the garden of the home he loved, and his casket had been lovingly painted with pictures by his many grandchildren. Friends and neighbours gathered in the sun, with the sea that he was so at home on at our backs and the song of birds in the air. Stories were shared. It was a joyful celebration of a man beloved by many.

Māori have been doing this for centuries with tangi. The dead are, and remain, important in te ao Māori, and the word tangi means 'to weep' and 'to sing a lament for the dead'. Those who have gone before are always part of gatherings through karanga, whaikōrero and mihi or pepeha. Tūpuna are an integral part of life, and remembering them is a way of sustaining their importance and the relationships with them. A tangi generally takes three days, and in that time stories, songs and speeches are shared. On the final day, there is usually a service led by a tohunga, and the body is taken to the urupā or cemetery for burial. Urupā are tapu, so at the entrance most have a water container or tap for mourners to wash their hands as they leave.

Janet Mikkelsen, a funeral director at Auckland's Aroha Funerals, works with a number of Māori and Pasifika families, and says that, 'Death is seen as a normal part of life. The coffin is open, there are children running around, visitors are welcomed.' Janet is of Irish Catholic heritage, and notes that for the Irish, too, the wake has always been seen as an important part of the process. 'We need to reclaim some of that and realise that it's healthy,' she says. Western cultures are slowly learning the benefits of a period of open mourning. Here in Aotearoa, Pākehā have absorbed some of the grace of the tangi, with families taking their loved ones home to farewell them.

Whichever way you choose to acknowledge the passing of a loved one, I have found that the process of saying goodbye is profoundly healing. Try not to rush it. Make a point of remembering the richness of the life led, the simple joys that the person brought you. As Mitch Albom noted in *Tuesdays with Morrie*, 'Death ends a life, not a relationship.'

At my mum's funeral, we read the following excerpt from *The Prophet* by the poet Kahlil Gibran. It was one of my mum's favourites.

> *What is it to die but to stand naked in the wind and to*
>   *melt into the sun?*
> *And what is it to cease breathing, but to free the breath*
>   *from its restless tides, that it may rise and expand*
>   *and seek God unencumbered?*
> *Only when you drink from the river of silence shall you*
>   *indeed sing.*
> *And when you have reached the mountain top, then you*
>   *shall begin to climb.*
> *And when the earth shall claim your limbs, then shall you*
>   *truly dance.*

Donating your body

In 2021, just 66 people in New Zealand donated organs. Those 66 people helped 191 others receive life-saving kidney, liver, lung, heart or pancreas transplants.

Imagine how many people could benefit if we all thought about organ donation. Of course, very few of us will be eligible to donate – less than one per cent of all New Zealanders die in a way that allows them to be organ donors. Organ donation is only possible when you die in intensive care on a ventilator, usually with devastating brain damage. Your organs will need to be removed by surgical teams within a few hours, and as Organ Donation New Zealand explains, 'This is a respectful process, carried out with care, using normal operating procedures.'

You can be an organ donor until you reach 80. Corneas can be donated up to 85. Eyes, brains, heart valves and skin can be donated after death without the need to be in hospital. If you're thinking about becoming a donor, check out the Organ Donation New Zealand website (donor.co.nz).

You might also consider donating your body to medical research. This is the ultimate gift to humankind. The medical schools at Auckland and Otago universities currently run Human Body Bequest programmes. Check with them before you make plans, because sometimes they are not able to take the body.

15

HEARTACHE
Grief

'Grief is the price we pay for love.'

—**Mary Ridpath Mann, *The Unofficial Secretary***

My mum and dad fell in love at first sight. They met in Lincolnshire in England, just before the outbreak of the Second World War. Dad was a young Kiwi, far from home, training with the Royal Air Force, and Mum was a ballet dancer who had turned to teaching dance because her father didn't want his eldest daughter 'on the stage'.

It was Christmas Eve, and the countryside was blanketed in snow. Dad was casually leaning against the mantelpiece in the house where he was billeted with his fellow airmen, sipping whisky by the roaring fire and trading tales of aeronautical exploits. Then Dinny Franks entered the room, and she and Ian Morrison locked eyes. Three weeks later they were engaged. It was the autumn of

1938, just as tensions were building in Europe. Dad would soon be called back home to fly for the RNZAF and Mum loved that airman enough to follow him across the world in 1941. My mother left her family and all she knew behind, and she never saw her father again – he died during the early stages of the war.

My parents' marriage lasted just short of 60 years. They were inseparable … and then they weren't. Dad died quite suddenly. They'd been on a cruise to Fiji. He came home with a cold which rapidly turned to pneumonia. Two days later he was gone. He was 84.

My mother was bereft. She gathered herself with the stoicism of her generation, helping us organise his funeral and painstakingly writing to all those who sent cards and flowers. Then she settled into her grieving.

By this time, she and Dad had already moved to a retirement village in Auckland. Dad had known he had a dicky heart and that his days were most likely numbered. He'd wanted Mum to be close to us. They'd made new friends quickly, so Mum was not alone. And yet she was *so* alone. I remember dropping in to visit her one afternoon and finding her sitting next to his empty chair, the tears coursing down her cheeks in despair.

It is a terrible pain when you lose someone you love, especially when that person is like the other half of you. And it can be the littlest things that set you off. As Frances told me, 'It's the music that does it to me. The songs we both loved.' When she lost her husband, Vic, they'd been married for 63 years. The pair had met at high school. 'I would rather have gone first,' Frances told me simply. 'The grief doesn't get any easier.'

Most married people who reach 85 will be widowed – the latest statistics show that the average life span for men in New Zealand is 79.5 years, while women tend to last a little longer, to 83.2 years. I often think of my mum weeping softly as she sat next to Dad's empty chair and, as I make my way through my seventies, I wonder what's in store for me and how I might manage if I am left alone as she was.

Talk about it

Grief is an inevitable part of life, particularly as we age, particularly if we love deeply. And yet so often we are afraid to talk about it. But talking about it helps us manage it, even though it never goes away.

My own grieving for Dad was intense at first. He was my rock, the whole family's rock. A wise head in times of uncertainty. I had long dreaded the thought of losing him. I knew he was not going to last forever. I cried when I found one of his big white linen hankies in my drawer. I used to love those soft hankies when I had a cold. He would always produce one for me when I cried as a child, proceeding to 'collect the tears' and put them in the breast pocket of the old wartime service shirts he was so fond of wearing on the weekends. He called it his 'fairy pocket'. I was filled with regret for the questions I hadn't asked him and the time I hadn't spent with him. But, eventually, I was able to look back and be thankful for his life, grateful for the laughter we shared and the encouragement he gave. I talk to him still.

Fortunately for Mum, our funeral director put us in touch with a grief counsellor, who proved to be a wonderful support, a gentle ear and a sensitive shoulder to cry on. Often, parents are reluctant to burden their adult children with the weight of their grief, and I'm sure this was the case for Mum. She was used to the old British stiff upper lip. Keep calm and carry on. It didn't sit well with her to share her troubles. But having someone who listened, without judgement, helped Mum navigate those first rocky months of mourning.

It was when I first became involved with Harbour Hospice that I saw the real value in being able to talk through your grief with someone removed from the family circle, someone with no preconceptions or biases. A hospice nurse, Maureen Frayling, who specialised in grief counselling for patients and their families, was finding it impossible to meet the growing need for her services. So, in her typically determined and forthright way, she set about establishing a centre dedicated to the counselling of all forms of grief – and so, the Grief Centre was born. I'm proud to be a patron of this wonderful organisation, too, and I cannot recommend it highly enough. (For more information, visit griefcentre.org.nz.)

It was Maureen who taught me that unresolved grief can cause us all sorts of problems down the track, perhaps without us realising it. Unresolved grief can impact on our physical health, digestion, sleep and energy levels. It can produce body aches and headaches and sighing. But it can also impact on our relationships and our ability to carry on with a fulfilling life. Of course, many people can manage their grief without the help of counselling, but many can't and, though they may have found it difficult to ask for help at first, they are inevitably glad they did.

When my good friend Gilly first told me her husband, Francis, had a brain tumour, it was a terrible shock. They were our oldest friends. We holidayed together for more than 40 years, and they're our eldest son, James's, godparents. In turn, we and James are godparents to their girls. We were very close. That cancer ended up taking Francis's life six years ago, leaving Gilly and her daughters, Matilda and Josie, behind. They have all been incredibly strong, forging on with their lives in exactly the way Francis would have wanted. But, as Gilly told me, 'Dealing with the grief was overwhelming. I found I had to accept help. No, not had to – I wanted to accept it. This was the most serious thing that had ever happened to me … How could I do this by myself?'

As Gilly says, she could feel the support and kindness of others. She knew they wanted to help. 'Family, friends, neighbours, workmates and my whole community felt the sadness, too,' she says. 'They wanted to do something positive that might make my day a little bit better. So I determined early on to let that happen. I wanted to accept that kindness and thoughtfulness. The alternative looked very bleak.'

She also found Lucy Hone's book *Resilient Grieving* (previously published as *What Abi Taught Us*) enormously helpful. 'It still is,' she says. Three central ideas from the book have stuck with Gilly. The first is, 'Don't lose what you have to what you have lost.' As Gilly explains, 'I liked this right off the bat. It kept me in touch with the importance of the present, and not making things even worse than they already were.'

The second is the title of the book. 'Resilient grieving. It is absolutely my watchword,' Gilly says. 'To me, that means grieving fully for what you have lost, and the person you love so much, but still being positive and maintaining a way to survive through it somehow, alongside the memories. So you are not diminishing the loss, but not letting it shape your life.' This was incredibly important to Gilly, especially as her daughters were only 18 and 14 at the time Francis died. 'I was very sure that I did not want them to be so affected by losing their father that it had a negative impact on them later in life,' Gilly says. 'The last thing he would have wanted was for us to fall apart, to not carry on with the things we loved to do, for the girls to not reach their potential.' She went on to do an amazing job raising her girls on her own. Matilda is now 25, a software engineer and qualified ski instructor. Josie is 21 with a bachelor of science and has qualified to work as a ski patroller, helping with medical emergencies on the ski field.

The third idea that Gilly found helpful was the chapter titled 'Positive Emotions'. In it, Hone states, 'It is well known that negative emotions abound in grief; we're looking to balance them out with some of the positive emotions, too.' This seemed right to Gilly. 'It really helps to have positive feelings around you,' she explains, 'and you can find them with a little bit of guidance. I focused on love, humour, gratitude, finding the awe in life – often in nature, and by remaining curious about all sorts of things.'

One other significant source of support for Gilly came in the form of hospice. Francis, and by extension Gilly, had spent a good deal of time supported by Dove Hospice so, as Gilly says, 'that organisation and the amazing people who work for them were easy for me to continue to talk to'. As she explains, they had a totally holistic attitude to the whole family, and offered all kinds of treatments, including healing massage, personal therapy, groups to talk to, and also a lounge where you could go and have a cup of tea and read the paper. 'I found this truly incredible,' Gilly says. 'For a year I went regularly to some of these sessions and I found comfort and a way to get through another day or week.'

My friend Deb, whom I spoke about in an earlier chapter, died in a hospice. Even though she'd been a nurse specialising in the care of older people, she had been adamant that she did not want to go to a hospice. She strove valiantly to stay at home and her husband, Paul, and wide group of friends rallied to help her. Paul, in particular, carried an enormous load. Deb seldom slept at night, so he would be up at all hours turning her, helping her to the toilet, comforting her. It took a toll on him, and on Deb, too. Eventually the decision was made to contact the local hospice, and the relief for both of them was enormous. Deb had instant access to the best possible palliative care, while Paul was able to rest and give his all to his beloved wife in her last days.

Going through it

Counsellors will tell you grief is messy. It's backwards and forwards and up and down. There is no timeframe.

Many will have heard of Elisabeth Kübler-Ross's five stages of grief: denial, anger, bargaining, depression and acceptance. Unfortunately, over time these stages became etched in stone, and misrepresented as some kind of list that one moved through systematically. The crucial thing many overlook is that Kübler-Ross described these stages as being experienced by the *dying* (not the grieving), and has since clarified that the idea was neither that people move through them in a linear fashion nor even experience all of them.

The truth is that grief is not something we process, go through and get over. It is a normal human response, and the experience of it will differ from person to person. You need to know you're not weak or going nuts because you hear your dead partner's voice or become prone to breaking down in tears at the drop of a hat. One of the great myths we need to shift is that you 'have to get over it'. That is just not a reality.

There are many theories about grief, but common to all is the need to 'hold the pain' – acknowledge it – and find meaning in life going forward. Grief researcher William Worden has outlined four stages, which you might find helpful.

1. Accept the reality of the loss

Initially there is the funeral ritual and learning to speak of the person in the past tense, so on one level the bereaved may have accepted the reality of the loss. However, they may be having trouble accepting the true impact of the loss in their daily lives, and that is painful.

2. Work through the pain

Each person is different. They may have to work through a range of emotions – sadness, fear, loneliness, despair, anger, guilt, regret, blame. It's important to acknowledge these feelings. Don't deny them. All these things need to be felt and examined.

3. Adjust to the environment from which the person is missing

This is especially difficult for people who have been in long-term relationships. It's a huge shock, and can result in a serious loss of confidence. 'Learning to live by yourself is hard,' Gilly says. 'I have never lived by myself before, so it is not a natural state for me. Like so many other people, the coincidence of losing a partner, children leaving home, and then stopping working all happened close together.'

In Mum's case, she was so used to doing things as a couple that she found it difficult to venture out alone. In essence, she had to 'find' herself. The loss of a long-term partner also often means having to learn a whole new range of skills: dealing with cooking, housework, maintenance, bills, finances and making big decisions alone. In time, Mum did find herself. She found great joy in new friendships and most especially in her great-grandchildren.

As for Gilly, planning has become a necessity. 'Planning events has always been part of my life, professionally and privately,' she says. 'Now, it's the way I survive. It means there is structure, a list, a schedule. I know my family and friends will laugh if they read this, but it is my way of giving myself a map, finding my way and discovering new pathways.'

4. Find an enduring connection with the person you've lost while making a 'different' life

Remember, your loved one lives on in your heart and mind. You carry them through life with you, in the form of memories and stories and precious times spent together. As your life changes and becomes a 'different' life, you can bring them with you by:

- talking about them
- sharing stories with those who knew them well
- carrying or wearing something precious that belonged to them
- celebrating their life
- creating new rituals and traditions to remember them.

Play the music you enjoyed together, have photos around, talk to them, sing the songs you both loved. Choose to survive and thrive, and at the same time acknowledge the discomfort.

As American research professor of social work and author Brené Brown says, 'When we get to own our story, we get to write "the end". Think, "I can choose to live on and find meaningful ways to live my life."'

Growth is possible

Grief counsellors tell me that although the pain will always be there, the context gets bigger. I have found this to be true. The world expands so that, in comparison, the grief becomes smaller. You continue to feel the sadness, but it's not as overwhelming.

Remember, love transcends death. It lives on beyond death. And growth is possible as an outcome of loss.

It may sound odd, but I often talk to my dad when I have a problem. As I said, he was wise, and I often sought his counsel when he was around. Many's the time I consider decisions I have to make and wonder what he would have done. And sometimes it's just the little things I call on him for, like finding me a spot in a carpark! 'Come on, Dad, there has to be one for me somewhere here,' I'll mutter under my breath. And, sure enough, one generally appears!

Sometimes grief can catch you unaware. A friend told me he was working at home one day when he noticed a rose blooming outside his window. It was coral, his mother's favourite colour. A wave of sadness flowed over him as he remembered her. He walked out into the garden and picked the rose and put it in a vase on his desk. A symbol of the continuing bond between mother and son.

There is one piece of advice for the grieving that really resonates with me. If you find you're overwhelmed, break your life down into 20-minute portions. When you wake, get up and think, 'What can I do for me?' Be present with what you need right now. Breaking life into moments just seems more manageable, even if the task you have in mind is daunting. Just do 20 minutes' worth.

When it comes to grief, it's difficult to categorise what is 'normal' and what is 'problematic'. There are, however, a few instances where grief can become a concern:

- if the survivor loses interest in work and socialising for a long period of time
- if there are distressing memories and longing for the dead person on a daily basis, over a long period of time
- if the survivor is having difficulty acknowledging that the person is dead, and they are avoiding reminders of that person, such as certain rooms, people or activities.

Sometimes, the one left behind may even develop symptoms similar to the ones experienced by their loved one, or psychosomatic symptoms like headaches and pains that can't be explained by physical problems.

Telling grief and depression apart is often difficult. However, depression tends to present with a long period of lethargy and fatigue, and a loss of interest in any outside activity. Grief, on the other hand, will allow moments of relief, peace and happiness. Glimmers of light are there.

Helping others

When someone you know is grieving, the most important thing you can do is lend an ear. Listen. Walk alongside them, garden together, have a coffee, walk along the beach or through the bush.

Check in regularly. There is often a flurry of concern and attention around the time of the death and funeral, and then it peters out. Be there for that lonely time when others have moved on with their lives.

Allow the person to talk about the deceased. Ask about the person, the little things that made them special.

And allow the grieving person to be free with their emotions. Let them cry, rage and weep in despair. Let them talk about their fear and guilt.

Just listen.

Grieving people don't want pity. Nor are they likely to respond if you say, 'Is there anything I can do?' or 'Just call me if you need me.' Be specific in your offers of help: 'I'm having a coffee, how about joining me?' or 'We're going for a walk on the beach, do you feel like coming?' or 'Want to go see a movie?'

Grieving people want to talk. They don't necessarily want 'solutions'. Be brave, open the conversation and then hunker down to listen. Try not to ask that open-ended 'How are you?' Sometimes that's too much to answer. Instead, maybe try, 'How are you feeling today, right now?'

Loss upon loss

We lost Mum when she was 94. She had developed Parkinson's in her late seventies, and it was in the latter stages of that disease that dementia began to attack her brain. It was a long, hard road to travel, both for her and for us children. It is never easy to parent your parent. It feels unnatural and just plain wrong.

I grieved for Mum long before she died. I grieved for her loss of independence, the loss of her ability to move. It was a terrible fate for someone who loved to dance. And, eventually, I grieved for the loss of her mind. It was quite a journey.

Fiercely independent, Mum stayed in her little house at the retirement village as long as possible. She loved that home and the memories it held of Dad. She was particularly attached to the rose garden he'd planted, and she loved to sit out in the garden and watch it bloom. (It's a delight to know it's blooming still.)

Soon though, it became clear that she needed full-time care, so she had to move to a nearby rest home that provided hospital care. The move to a rest home or hospital is, in many ways, a social death, and a period of grieving almost inevitably follows. A person becomes resigned to being there. They can feel unwanted, of no use. Life is no longer meaningful. They have no purpose. The person can feel powerless when decisions are made about their care, and those decisions can be hard to process.

Few people enter a rest home because they want to. It's usually something beyond their control that forces the issue. A question here: if you decide to place your parent or loved one in a rest home, are you making that decision for them or for you? If you make it because you are concerned for their safety, because they really need help and can no longer make decisions for themselves, then it is probably a good choice. If, however, you make it because you won't have to make contact so often, because you can't be bothered to deal with their 'issues', or because you want to control their life, then perhaps you should rethink.

The loss of independence is one of the most painful losses to suffer, and one Mum struggled with. It often begins with the loss of the ability to drive. It may seem like just yesterday that you were champing at the bit to get your licence as a teenager; suddenly, in what feels like the blink of an eye, a lifetime of achievement and challenge counts for nothing. This is the end. No more licence. Self-esteem plummets.

Mum began to see herself as a burden. In the rest home, she had little choice about simple, everyday tasks we all take for granted. She had to shower when there was someone there to help, she had to eat what was on offer, there was no avocado on toast, no bacon and eggs for dinner just because she felt like it. Small freedoms were sacrificed. Even laundry was institutional. Mum's beautiful delicate nighties were tossed in with old socks and trousers and came back grey and torn. Everything had to have a name tag, just like boarding school. Precious jewellery could no longer be worn, 'just in case'.

For Mum, the loss of her home and possessions was a source of deep sadness. Gone was the furniture that had been in the family for generations, the special things that were a link to Dad and us children. We did manage to furnish her room with a few special pieces, and my siblings and I held on to sentimental items so she could see them in our homes.

What's more, visits from friends and neighbours became intermittent ... then dropped away entirely. Even a long-trusted doctor was not able to treat her in the rest home.

So many losses.

Anger is one of the most common reactions to loss. It can override every other feeling – sadness, loneliness, hurt, guilt. People who are feeling angry will often blame others, especially the ones closest to them who are helping them the most.

How best, then, to help someone you love navigate those feelings that accompany a move into care?

Again, by listening. In particular, there are a few things it helps to remember:

- **Let them voice their feelings.** Often people in care will say, 'I wish I could die,' or 'I'm tired of living. I want to go.' It's hard to hear, but trying to prevent them from saying those things will only cause them to turn their feelings inward. They need to be able to give vent to how they are feeling, so they can process those emotions and relieve the pressure and sadness. A good listener will allow these thoughts to be voiced, simply sitting there and maybe even acknowledging things by saying something like, 'I understand you're feeling really sad.'
- **Be patient.** People going through this transition to rest-home care may feel the need to repeat the story of their losses time and time again. Just listen.
- **Allow time travel.** Rest-home residents will often use regression to cope. In this way, they can return to a safe place. Many older people return to the time when they were children, and they may become so involved in that time that they use the names of people from their past and apply them to the living. Let them.
- **Put words to fear.** They may be afraid. Encourage them to express their fears aloud. Help them to find someone who can be supportive when they're frightened.

The more love and care you can give your parent or loved one, the easier it will be for them and for you.

Walk with them on this journey, and try not to judge.

There is no 'normal'

Everyone experiences loss in different ways. Do you tend to seek out support? Or do you tend to internalise and limit your connections with others? Are you generally a positive thinker? Do you have a strong faith? How is your self-esteem? The answers to all these questions will colour the way each person responds to grief.

Grief counsellor Johann van den Berg's mum grew up and got married in South Africa, and when his dad died she said, 'I just want to be in there with him,' as she gazed at his coffin. Afterwards, she remained at home with the dog for a number of years, then spent five years in a rest home. 'All she wanted to take to the rest home were two landscapes of Africa and pictures of Dad and the dog,' Johann says. When things are dire, he explains, we home in on the things that are really important in our lives.

It's crucial to have lots of conversations about and tangible reminders of lives lived together – a ring, a rose, a picture of a dog. As you get older, you focus more closely on the things that really matter to you, that have helped define your relationships – things to carry forward, memories of your homeland, the place you feel most connected to. We should, Johann says, 'tap into our lived experience. We don't do it as much as we should. It gives us more meaning and hope. Ask: who am I? Where have I come from? What's meaningful for me?'

As we age, grief comes to us in many forms. Some studies have found that having the ability to anticipate loss leads to an easier grief experience. Other studies, however, find there's no relation between a time of anticipation and the severity of grief once a person has died. Clinical psychologist Therese Rando specialises in grief and loss, and has written many books on the subject. Her work on anticipatory grief, in particular, shows that this form of grief is experienced from two distinct perspectives: from that of the dying individual, and that of all those who care about them.

Anticipatory grief is the grief you may feel in the days, months or even years before a terminally ill loved one dies. According to Allison Werner-Lin, a licensed clinical social worker and associate professor at the University of Pennsylvania, 'It's the experience of knowing that a change is coming, and starting to experience bereavement in the face of that.' It's not a way of getting 'through' the grieving process before a person dies; rather, it's that the shock of death is removed. The death is predictable, expected. Not everyone will have the capacity for anticipatory grief; having time before death does not automatically mean people can actively process emotions related to an impending loss. Again, it is different for everyone. It's reassuring, however, to know that it is possible to give up the hope of a future together and grieve for that, while still caring in the present for a dying loved one.

The most common concern about anticipatory grief is that it can result in a premature separation or detachment from the dying person, who may then feel abandoned. Additionally, the stress of caring for a person who's dying can, when added to the anticipatory grief already experienced, lead to emotional numbness at the actual time of death. It may even cause you to question your love for the deceased.

'Anticipatory grief is more than post-death grief stretched out,' Rando says. 'It's a journey to the ultimate loss, but is composed of many losses: the past, present and future.' And, as she explains, it can be especially complicated in a family setting, 'because each member of the family will be grieving in their own way and in their own time'. Some, she points out, may not have begun the grieving process while others have already started to separate themselves emotionally from the person who's dying.

At the end of the day, remember this: no one should be telling you how to grieve.

Each of us has our own way and will do it in our own time.

16

RIDING THE WAVE
Resilience

'You have power over your mind – not outside events.
Realise this and you will find strength.'
—Marcus Aurelius

Change is stressful. I'm definitely not good with it. Same job for nearly 40 years, same house for more than 40, not to mention same husband for 50 plus!

When Chris and I were first married, we lived in his hometown, Christchurch. That's where we met. We were both working for what was then the New Zealand Broadcasting Corporation, but when he was shoulder-tapped for a job in Auckland, I became a reluctant follower. I was perfectly content in Christchurch. We'd bought a little two-bedroom bungalow in St Albans, my job in the Christchurch newsroom was going well and we had a great group of friends. But Chris was keen to develop his career, and it looked as though much of the action would be in Auckland. So, we packed up my little Morris Minor with all we could carry and drove north, complete with the maidenhair fern hanging out the window!

For six months, I was miserable. I missed my mates, I missed the house and garden we'd left behind, I missed the daffodils in Christchurch's parks, I missed being able to see the mountains. I'd found a job in what was then the South Pacific Television newsroom, but I felt rattled and rootless. I wasn't sure where we were heading.

Those same feelings can come with any significant life change. The change that comes with retirement is a biggie, but there are also other momentous changes as we age. We may lose some of our dearest friends, we may become ill or we may have to learn to live with a disability. We may decide to downsize, which will involve getting rid of many of our treasured possessions. We may move towns and have to adapt to a whole new way of life. As mentioned earlier, we may even lose our driver's licence – and this last one is an especially potent source of anxiety and depression in older people. All the older people I spoke to when researching this book ranked losing their driver's licence as one of their biggest fears about ageing. Suddenly you lose your independence. You become 'dependent', either on public transport or on someone else to help you get around. That loss of independence is a huge hurdle to cross. Chris and I had a rude awakening just the other day when we tried to book a rental car for an upcoming trip to the UK and discovered that you're charged a surcharge if you're over 65. Good grief. That's barely past middle age! What are they thinking? I bet I'm a better driver now than I was in my twenties or thirties …

All in all, it can feel as though life is closing early.

Little wonder, in times of such huge change and adjustment, that anxiety, stress and depression often come calling. While feeling out of sorts and lost is perfectly normal, some of us end up feeling these things more acutely and for longer.

Toxic ageism

It doesn't help that everyone and everything around us suddenly starts writing us off because of ageist stereotypes. While ageism is also targeted at the young, it has particularly damaging effects on the health and well-being of older people.

Whenever I've asked others to tell me about their own experiences of ageism, the same examples pop up. Other people telling them, 'You look good for your age!' Many express the feeling that, because they're now old, they need to 'keep up or get out of the way'. Many people worry about weighing others down. Many others report, 'It hurts when people see purely my age.'

My lovely friend Stella recently went into a chemist to pick up a prescription. She had two scripts to collect – one for her ears and one for her eyes. The young shop assistant took one glance at her and began to talk very LOUDLY and SLOWLY, looking Stella straight in the eyes, 'Now THIS one is for your EARS and THIS one is for your EYES.' Stella, who is thoroughly intelligent and energetic, was a bit bemused. It wasn't until she left the chemist that she suddenly realised, with horror, 'Oh my goodness! She thinks I'm senile!' It was one of those watershed moments.

There are all kinds of negative stereotypes about 'old people' out there. That the old should pass on power to the young. That the old shouldn't consume too many resources. That the old should not engage in activities seen as being purely for the young. All this can become a self-fulfilling prophecy and really affect how older people see themselves.

Ageism doesn't just come from individual people, either. It's present in society's structures as a whole. Take the move by banks and post offices to close local branches and shift their businesses online, for example. This has caused problems for so many older people, particularly those in the 80+ age group, who may not have had as much exposure to computers over their lifetime. It makes their ability to access basic services significantly more difficult, which only adds to the feeling of being shut out and written off by the rest of society. Even with those organisations offering one-on-one help, sometimes it's just a step too far for many older people.

While the whole world of technology may be overwhelming for some, most older people are perfectly capable of mastering it. They just need a little time, patience and consideration. A plea here from all older people to their tech-savvy relatives: by all means show me, but please DON'T DO IT FOR ME!

So many of the older people I spoke to for this book mentioned tech problems – phones that aren't designed for arthritic fingers, technical language that may as well be Greek, inaccessible and hard-to-navigate websites.

The World Health Organization has identified three strategies to reduce ageism that have a proven track record:

1. Address it in the law and in policy documents.
2. Teach the public about its effects, and how to combat it, through public education campaigns.
3. Enable intergenerational contact in all areas of society.

That last one's probably the most important, because ageism starts in childhood, when children pick up subtle and sometimes not-so-subtle cues about ageist stereotypes and prejudices. No one is born ageist. We are just constantly fed negative messages about ageing, such as 'It's sad to be old.'

Anxiety

Scottish Baptist minister Alexander Maclaren, who died in 1910, apparently said, 'Our anxiety does not empty tomorrow of its sorrows, but only empties today of its strengths.' That really resonates with me. How right he was!

It's common to become more anxious as we age. According to Anxiety New Zealand, the most common fears in older people have to do with falling (particularly if you've had a previous fall), becoming dependent on others, being left alone, facing housing and financial worries, and illness and death. Those are all pretty big worries, and they all come with age.

Anxiety as a condition, however, is a little different from just feeling a bit worried about things from time to time. It's often characterised by racing thoughts, constant worrying, a sense of hopelessness and feeling a bit 'out of control'. People suffering anxiety can be guilty of black-and-white thinking – they have a tendency to see only the extremes of a situation. They might take others' actions or words completely out of context, letting them take on monstrous proportions and imagining slights where there are none. In other words, you might be busy thinking you *know* what others are thinking (usually something terrible about you), but you're way off beam!

We all experience a bit of anxiety every now and then. It's a natural response to being scared or feeling threatened. However, the precise quality of the anxiety you experience will vary depending on all kinds of factors, including the situation you're in and also your own personality. Experts sometimes distinguish between state anxiety and trait anxiety. The former tends to show up when you face a potential threat – you may feel your heart beating faster and your mind clouded by worry – but it passes as soon as the threat does. Trait anxiety, by comparison, is more of a fixed part of your personality.

If you're more prone to trait anxiety, you're more likely to feel threatened by specific situations or even by the world in general than a person less prone to it. This form of anxiety has an unhelpful tendency to pop up in everyday situations, especially those that might not be immediately worrisome or terrifying to others. It's characterised by overthinking and creating false negative scenarios. Haven't heard from your editor? They must hate the article! Your partner seems a bit stand-offish? They must want to leave you! Your friend hasn't called you back since you left a message this morning? They must not like you anymore!

People with trait anxiety may also see social threats where there are none, and can become anxious about meeting new people or going to new places. This form of anxiety can affect your sleep and your ability to concentrate. You may become irritable, and your heart may race.

Cognitive behaviour therapy (see page 127) can help with trait anxiety. There's also a tactic I employ whenever I notice myself thinking negatively. Say I have a particularly scary audience to present to – perhaps one made up of my peers (the scariest!). Usually, I tend to start thinking, 'They'll all see through me. I'm not deserving of their attention. They'll be judging me.' I try to notice those feelings, and then I try to turn them around. I visualise the presentation. I tell myself that my content is good – it's interesting and relevant – and then I imagine the audience listening with rapt attention and giving me long applause when I've finished. I imagine how I'll feel at the end of it, when it has gone well, and all the satisfaction that goes with that. Sometimes it works, sometimes it doesn't, but it's well worth a try!

Stress

One night towards the end of my time presenting the news at TVNZ, I was halfway through the bulletin when the autocue suddenly became a black hole. There were no words. I could still see the studio and the people around me; it was just the cue that had gone blank. No matter how much I blinked, I couldn't make the words reappear.

It was scary. My heart was pounding, my skin sweaty. It lasted for around 30 seconds – a long time on live television! – and then everything righted itself.

Of course I was anxious about whether it would happen again … and it did, several times on different nights. I began memorising the scripts in case I blanked out again, and of course that only made me more anxious.

I was convinced something was seriously wrong. My doctor sent me to a neurologist, and scans were done, but there was nothing to see. It was a particularly stressful period at work for me, so that's what it was put down to: stress.

Stress is the silent killer. It can manifest physically as headaches, an upset stomach and back pain, and it can affect pretty much every part of your life, from relationships to work, leisure and sleep. It plays a big part in the incidence of major diseases like heart issues, high blood pressure and diabetes. While the link between chronic stress and cancer is deemed 'not clear' by the US National Institute of Health and Cancer Research UK, stress can nonetheless alter the levels of certain hormones in the body and put you at greater risk of developing cancer. In fact, it's estimated more than 80 per cent of doctors' visits are caused by stress-related illness. Daily agitation is a fact of life in this busy world of ours. I notice it especially while sitting in traffic if I'm running late. I can literally feel the cortisol levels rising.

When you're angry or stressed, the brain is flooded with adrenaline, noradrenaline and cortisol. This raises the heart rate, tenses the muscles and sets off the fight-or-flight response. Normal blood pressure is around 120/80, but when we're stressed that can rise to as much as 220/130, increasing the risk of a heart attack or stroke.

Back when my autocue kept disappearing, I had heard about Transcendental Meditation (TM). A lot of people in my line of work did it. And I figured that if it was good enough for the likes of Tom Hanks, Oprah Winfrey, Rupert Murdoch and Sir Paul McCartney, it was probably good enough for me. I decided to give it a go.

One of the reasons TM appealed was you could do it anywhere – in the car, at the beach, on a plane – so long as you could sit and close your eyes. You don't have to cross your legs or assume any pose. You don't have to chant. TM is a form of silent meditation where you use a mantra given to you by your teacher. My mantra is a Sanskrit word, and it is mine alone. I think it silently to myself, and it's a way of gently bringing focus back to the meditation. The aim is to reach a deep calm and silence in the mind.

The breath is not important with TM. You just sit and breathe normally, and gently begin repeating your mantra in your head. I usually find as I continue to meditate that my breath becomes shallower, and I become aware of sounds around me – cars passing, birdsong, the wind in the trees. The important thing is not to force anything. Thoughts come and go. Sometimes, especially when you are learning to meditate, you will feel your meditation is wall-to-wall thought. That's OK. Let the thoughts come, acknowledge them, and then draw yourself gently back to your meditation.

To transcend is to 'go beyond'. TM is a way of going beyond thought to a state of total silence. Maharishi Mahesh Yogi, the Indian guru who developed and popularised the technique back in the 1960s and '70s, would often liken the mind to a lake. The ripples on top of the water are our conscious thoughts. As you go deeper into the lake, the ripples still, and you reach the subconscious.

With TM, the mind settles to stillness and the body rests deeply. The fight-or-flight response in the brain is switched off, and the mind–body balance is restored. In addition, serotonin (the happiness hormone) increases. So, what's not to like?

To me, TM is a tool for health and well-being. And I've found it to be one of the most important tools in my box. Added to that, my husband says I'm 'much easier to live with' when I'm meditating. Ha! That's a big endorsement!

There are many, many different types of meditation out there that spring from different cultures, religions and traditions. Find one that suits you and keep practising. Meditation is a skill that needs to be worked on – it's often likened to a muscle that needs exercising.

Here are a few tips that you may find helpful for any kind of meditation:

- **Start slow.** Maybe with five or ten minutes first thing in the morning. As you get better at it, you can build up to longer sessions.
- **Schedule it.** Try to meditate at roughly the same time every day.
- **Get comfortable.** Sit upright anywhere that's relaxing and quiet.
- **Focus on what you're feeling.** Don't try to suppress your thoughts. Let them come … and then gently bring yourself back to your meditation.

Here are some places you can find out more:

- Headspace app (headspace.com)
- Verywell Mind (go to verywellmind.com and search for 'meditation')
- *Greater Good Magazine* (go to greatergood.berkley.edu and search for 'meditation')
- Transcendental Meditation website (transcendentalmeditation.org.nz).

Try it … it's like taking a mental shower!

Depression

I have what my sister charitably calls a 'mercurial' personality. In between experiencing the regular ups and downs of life, I also experience great highs and great lows. It's a rollercoaster ride. I have from time to time become acquainted with the Black Dog, the first time post-natally after our first child was born, again after a serious bout of viral meningitis and to a lesser extent during that stressful period in the latter part of my time at TVNZ. I found it hard to get out of bed. I'd wake up feeling exhausted and jittery. I lost confidence in myself and retreated from contact with my friends. I was lonely, yet I didn't want to be around people. It was hard to see the joy in life.

Depression is not a normal part of ageing. Nor is it a sign of weakness or a character flaw. And you can't just 'snap out of it'. If you constantly feel tired and hopeless, if you're having trouble working, eating, sleeping or just plain functioning, and if that continues for a length of time, day after day, then you may have depression. Of course, these feelings can be triggered by significant life events – the death of a loved one, the sale of your family home or the transition to retirement, to name but a few. It's normal to feel dodgy about these changes, but many people will come right, given time. Depression is when those feelings last for a long period. That's when it's time to see your doctor for advice.

It's worth learning to recognise the signs, both in yourself and your loved ones. Seek help if you spot any of the following:

- a persistent sad, anxious or 'empty' mood
- a loss of interest in hobbies and activities
- feelings of hopelessness and pessimism
- feelings of guilt, worthlessness and helplessness
- decreased energy and fatigue
- difficulty concentrating, remembering and making decisions
- difficulty sleeping, including waking early or oversleeping
- appetite changes
- poor personal hygiene, such as not showering or shaving
- thoughts about suicide or death
- restlessness and irritability
- no interest in seeing loved ones
- aches and pains that have no clear physical cause and don't ease with treatment.

There are also a number of factors that increase your risk of depression:

- having a family history of depression
- misusing drugs or alcohol – seniors dealing with depression are at double the risk of developing an alcohol dependency
- experiencing stressful life events, such as death, divorce or caring for someone with a chronic disease
- being lonely or isolated
- sleeping poorly
- having a disability.

Former All Black Sir John Kirwan has done more for the awareness of depression and mental health here in New Zealand than a multitude of well-intentioned campaigns. He was crippled with anxiety at the height of his rugby career, and his courage and honesty about what he has been through has helped to change people's attitudes towards anxiety and depression. That we can now talk openly about our feelings is in large part thanks to him.

When he was suffering most, he says he felt out of control in his head. He completely lost confidence and was almost 'flatlining'. Anxiety attacks that took about two minutes felt like they lasted two days. 'Hardening up' was not an option. Medication helped, but John is also proactive about finding ways to stay well. He has discovered he's an 'active relaxer': he swims, cooks and seeks out the company of friends at his local café and market. He says mental wellness has come from slowing down and taking time to be kind to others. There's that social connection again! Little surprise that it's a profoundly protective factor for beating depression.

Depression, at its most sinister, is life-threatening. This is something Caroline Chevin knows all too well. In 2018, she lost her husband, the much loved and widely respected journalist Greg Boyed, to suicide. Two years later, she bravely spoke to journalist Zara Potts for the *New Zealand Herald* about that experience. 'I think we need to talk about depression more,' she said. 'I have had a lot of emails recently from people who have had severe depression and come through the worst of it, and I've also heard from people who have lost loved ones to depression, and I think it's time we started to talk more openly and honestly about this and try to take away some of the stigma attached to it.'

It's true that, while we have made great strides forward, we still have a long way to go in our understanding and acceptance of mental health conditions such as depression. One thing that struck me out of everything Chevin noted was her description of how Greg's depression manifested. 'He wasn't a typical sufferer of depression,' she said. 'We associate depression with a lack of vitality, someone who can't get up in the morning, someone who is sad and shows no interest in life – these are the signs we are told to look out for. But what if that person doesn't show any of these signs?' Greg, she said, was the opposite: 'energetic, he always went to work, he was always helping others'. 'That shows me how little we really know about this illness,' Chevin said. 'He had told me from the beginning of our relationship that he suffered from depression, but even though I knew this, I didn't know all the faces of this illness … I only realised the year that he died that these aspects of what I thought were his temperament, like moodiness and irritability, were actually signs of his illness.'

We often hear that those suffering the symptoms of depression should ask for help, but as Chevin pointed out, that becomes difficult when the sufferer is being up front about their condition … but hiding the extent to which it's affecting them. It's really hard to know that they need care when it seems like everything is OK. As Chevin noted, Greg was doing all the things he was 'supposed to do' – he exercised regularly, he talked to friends, he sought treatment. But, she went on, when someone's doing all those things and still not feeling any better, 'I think they then start to feel like they've failed. In theory, it's a good idea to ask people how they're feeling but, in reality, I don't think that's enough.'

So, what to do? Well, as with so many things, it seems all that any of us can do is our best. Keep an eye on yourself and on your loved ones. Remember, even if you or your loved one seem fine, you and they may still need a bit of support. And, above all else, please know it is a sign of strength to seek help, whether from family and friends or from a medical professional.

If you're on medication for depression, read as much as you can about your meds and ask your doctor lots of questions. Make sure you fully understand possible side effects and be careful about swapping brands or coming off medication suddenly.

You are not alone. There are many, many others on the same journey.

Building resilience

The past few years have been a long and bumpy ride for everyone. The Covid pandemic has affected everything. New variants keep appearing; just when we think we're out of the woods, cases begin to spike again. Lives have been lost. Jobs, too. Businesses are continuing to struggle. The cost of living is out of control. Wars in the Middle East and the Ukraine grind on relentlessly at the time of writing, and climate change is slapping us in the face. It feels as if the world has swung off its axis. It's been incredibly tough for so many.

Most recently here in New Zealand, the weather has devastated entire communities, claiming lives and leaving families homeless and without the jobs they've spent a lifetime creating. No matter what sort of life you've lived through these past years, you will have felt some anxiety and stress. It's been impossible to plan anything. We worry about our health, our jobs, our homes, our kids' jobs and their homes, our grandchildren, and so much more.

Most of all, though, we worry about the future. And all that worry and stress and anxiety takes a toll.

Constant negative thoughts are exhausting. The body feels what the mind thinks. Personally, I have little to worry about in the great scheme of things, but I've found myself feeling discombobulated these past pandemic years. I love that word. It sounds how I feel: bobbing about, directionless, anxious, untethered. It literally means bewildered, befuddled, thrown. Sound familiar?

If there's anything I have learnt over the years, it is that there's no quick fix for conditions like anxiety, stress and depression. Yes, often a course of antidepressants or anti-anxiety drugs can help to set you on the path to wellness. These drugs certainly have their place. But, as Caroline Chevin noted in that same interview with the *Otago Daily Times*, 'I think a lot of people see medication as being like a magic pill that will make everything better and, a lot of the time, it does help people but sometimes it doesn't. In many cases, you are treating the symptoms, rather than the cause.'

There are all kinds of things that can trigger or exacerbate mental illness: poverty, sickness, unemployment, your relationship falling apart, retirement or the death of a loved one. Pills won't be able to fix these things for you. It's also worth remembering that all medications can have side effects, and some are highly addictive. In the past when the Black Dog has been following me around and it's not a big dog – more of a chihuahua, all things considered – I've resisted being medicated. At one point, I did head to our family GP and he prescribed amitriptyline, which is often used to treat migraines, low mood and depression, but it left me feeling woolly-headed. I don't like taking pills at the best of times, although I'm grateful they're there for when you really need them. I am a great believer in giving natural remedies a try, too. Just make sure you check them out with your doctor first. And a big rider here: antidepressants have their place. Listen to your doctor. If you want to try coming off antidepressants, check with a medical expert first, then follow their advice. Don't just stop abruptly, as that can be dangerous.

If you're keen to try a natural approach, I've personally found ashwagandha root really helpful. Often called 'the crown jewel' of Ayurvedic medicine, it may help reduce stress and anxiety, decrease inflammation and aid sleep. Ayurveda is one of the world's oldest holistic healing practices. Developed in India more than 3000 years ago, it's based on the idea that good health depends on a balance between body, mind and spirit. Look for a product made from ashwagandha root (not the leaves) and, as always, consult your doctor first.

I'm not for a moment suggesting anyone throw away their prescription medicines. In general, they provide immense benefits, but we also live in a highly medicated society that suggests pills can fix any problem. When it comes to caring for your mental health as you get older, Auckland University professor Ngaire Kerse, a GP herself, says, 'We should be having more conversations about resilience in old age, the same way we talk about resilience in children and young adults.'

Resilience is the ability to cope and recover from setbacks. It allows you to respond to life's challenges and face them head on. Resilient people still feel emotions like fear, sadness, anxiety and anger, but they know that these feelings are temporary and can be dealt with until they pass. Resilient people are kind to themselves when times are hard. They are able to look at problems rationally and seek solutions. The more resilient you are, the faster you'll bounce back from life's curly ones.

So, how can you be more resilient?

If you're prone to anxiety, depression or stress, there are a number of things you can do to care for yourself and build resilience:

- **Keep track of how you're feeling.** Just make a brief note in your diary each day. By doing this, I've noticed my hormones have a huge effect on how I'm feeling (yes, I know – still, after all these years!), as do the phases of the moon, particularly on my sleep patterns. So, when I know I'm coming up to a hormonal time or the full moon, I try to schedule less in my day.

- **Say no.** It's taken me a while to learn to say 'no' when I'm overloaded, but it has been a great lesson. I used to feel guilty about it. Not anymore! For instance, I'm often asked to make speeches, but that's something that instantly gives me a knot in the stomach, sweaty palms and anxiety. I used to force myself to walk through the fire of public speaking, having read the book *Feel the Fear and Do It Anyway* (quite possibly written for me, to get me out of my comfort zone!), and I admit there is something to be said for that approach as I generally felt great afterwards. But now, I figure life's too short to be doing things you don't want to do! So, unless it's a cause I'm thoroughly invested in, it's generally a 'no'.

- **Nurture relationships.** Spend time cultivating your social networks. When you're depressed or anxious, it's very easy to withdraw from other people, but this is the very time you need to be with them. This is the time to 'feel the fear and do it anyway'! Even if I don't feel like seeing anyone, I push myself to make contact with friends and family, as chat is a tonic.

- **Keep well hydrated.** When you're dehydrated, the levels of cortisol rise in the body, causing you to feel more stressed. Try to keep water handy at all times.

- **Eat well.** When you're stressed, it's so easy to put yourself last. You may tend to skip meals or go for the fast-food option and you don't make time for exercise. Folate and vitamin B12 are mood improvers. You can find them in good old leafy greens like silver beet, kale and spinach, and they're also in pulses, wholegrains and fish.

- **Get out in nature.** Look at this stunning country of ours. Really look at it. Take your shoes off and ground yourself walking along a sandy beach or through a grassy field, paddle in a stream, listen to the birdsong. Take your earphones out and absorb the moment. Explore the bush.

- **Exercise!** Walk, run, dance, box, go to the gym, try yoga or Pilates – whatever you enjoy. If exercising is the last thing you want to do, do it anyway, because all the science tells us that exercise is good for the brain. It really doesn't have to involve a class of any sort. A brisk walk and a bit of stretching will do the trick. Being physically active releases a flood of feel-good endorphins in the brain. Soak them up!

- **Walk the dog (if you have one).** This has been one of my greatest stress-relievers. A dog gives you a great reason to get out of bed in the morning. They have to be walked, and what's more you meet other dog-walkers while you're out, so it can be a really social time for both of you. Dogs give you unconditional love and they're always happy to see you, especially if you have a treat in your pocket! Our Rhodesian ridgeback, Nala, is a big girl. It's like having a small horse in the house, but she's a great companion.

She's sitting beside me right now, in fact, happy on her bed, waiting patiently for me to take a break so she can have a walk.

- **Practise gratitude.** When you wake up, before you get out of bed, just take a moment to think of five things you're grateful for. There will be five, trust me, even on the bleakest of days.

- **Avoid comparison.** Try not to compare your life to that of others. We all have 'stuff' going on. Remember, 'Comparison is the thief of joy.'

- **Laugh!** Take in some stand-up comedy. I've even been known to linger in bookshops, chortling over hilarious birthday cards. There's a reason people practise laughter yoga!

- **Let things suck.** Sometimes, when I've tried everything else and it's just not working, I like to follow American author John Green's advice: 'I just give myself permission to suck … I find this hugely liberating!' So do I, John! Let's face it, all this striving for perfection can be bloody wearing and sometimes we just need to be OK with things sucking.

The final word here has to go to trust. Through it all, remember this: 'Trust yourself. The strength lies within.' (That one's all me!)

Cultivating happiness

I had the privilege of meeting the Dalai Lama, wise soul that he is, when he visited our local hospice some years ago. He is probably the most serenely positive person I've ever met, and he told me that happiness and peace lie within us all (then gave one of his hearty chuckles).

Of course, he was right. Happiness and peace do lie within us all. But how to find them?

I've already mentioned that studies have shown optimists tend to live longer, have fewer heart issues and don't suffer as much depression. We now know there is definitely a genetic link as to whether we tend to look on the bright side or not. Some people are literally wired to experience happiness. They're glass-half-full people. They have a positive outlook on life. No matter what happens, they look for the silver lining.

Having said that, your genes are only part of the story. Happiness can be a choice, too. It's something you can practise and encourage. Just remember, it is not possible to be happy 100 per cent of the time! And keep this thought, from a 2011 paper published by Berkeley University psychology professor Iris B. Mauss and colleagues, in mind: 'Those who seek happiness seem to have the most trouble actually gaining it.'

Happiness isn't so much to do with what we *have* as what we feel. It's characterised by a sense of contentment and satisfaction. Notably, when we're grateful for what we have, even if it's not as much as we want, and we focus on the things that aren't wrong in our lives, we're happier. When we feel grateful, the brain releases dopamine and serotonin. Commonly known as the 'feel-good' hormones, they help balance us out. It's all about employing that glass-half-full philosophy. Robert Emmons, a psychology professor at the University of California, Davis, has found that practising gratitude lowers your blood pressure, improves immunity and helps sleep. Gratitude is also associated with an increase in 'good' cholesterol and a decrease in 'bad' cholesterol.

Happiness is a by-product of leading a meaningful life, a life with a sense of purpose. This is something many of us already know instinctively. Soon after Ella Wilson's mother died in the 1918 flu pandemic, she was separated from her father and four brothers. Ella was four at the time. Speaking to the *Rotorua Daily Post* at the age of 107, she said it's important to 'count your blessings and get on with it'.

Her thoughts, looking back on her life? 'I always believed there was a pot of gold at the foot of the rainbow. I wondered when we would see it. But now I realise we had that pot of gold at our feet all the time.'

Don't lose sight of that pot of gold.

Finding peace

I'm not a church-goer. Nor were my parents, though both had a faith. Dad would read passages from *Good News for Modern Man* (the New Testament in modern English) every morning. The two of them lived following Christian principles and were keen for me not to be a 'heathen' – their word, not mine! They wanted some sort of religious instruction for me, so that's how I ended up spending my formative years at an Anglican boarding school in rural Rangitikei.

The school had its own beautiful little chapel. It smelt of candlewax, furniture polish and lilies. The whole school went to chapel twice a day, and three times on Saturdays – twice for services, and once to practise singing the hymns. I especially loved the singing, despite being pretty much tone-deaf. We would belt out the traditional versions of 'Jerusalem' and 'Praise, My Soul' while the sun shone softly through the stained-glass windows. It was a peaceful and lovely place, and every now and then there'd be a sermon that made you think, even as a teenager of the swinging '60s.

That little chapel gave me a sense of calm I still feel today whenever I enter a church, mostly for weddings or funerals. And that sense of calm is something I seek when I start feeling worried or depressed or stressed. It's how I try to find some peace within myself. I came away from boarding school believing in a higher power, so I have a sense that there is something greater than ourselves … although exactly what that something is, I haven't yet figured out.

In Pasifika communities, the church is very powerful. Life is anchored by religion. Every meeting begins with a prayer, and a form of mindfulness is practised – being grateful for what you have, not dwelling on what you don't have. With church comes a sense of belonging. Friendships are made. Help is given. People notice absences. 'Where is John?' 'Oh, he's had a fall. We should take him some food.' Pasifika elders I spoke to for this book told me that church, for them, is often the happiest place to be. It's social, and it's where they find a sense of peace.

Similarly, the famously long-lived Loma Linda Adventists see God as a positive influence, someone they can communicate with and gain comfort from. They have fewer problems with depression than those who have no spiritual connection.

A number of studies have linked participation in religion to longevity. Ohio State University researchers found that those with a religious affiliation lived as much as nine years longer than others. However, as the researchers were quick to point out, that could have been because belonging to a church can mean you're more socially engaged, less lonely, and less likely to be abusing drugs or alcohol. What's more, you're probably praying or meditating on a regular basis, and therefore reducing your stress.

Interestingly, the Harvard Study of Adult Development found that spirituality or religious adherence had little association with healthy ageing. Instead, the study found it was hope and love that made the difference. George Vaillant, a former director of the study, remarked that ageing allows us time to experience spirituality. Time to smell the roses, if you like. It increases the time we have to be internally quiet. Age focuses us and, hopefully, grounds us.

As you age, it's worth finding that place or thing that gives you a sense of peace. It doesn't have to be mainstream religion. It could be any of the things suggested in this chapter – laughing, walking in nature, meditating – or something of your own choosing. What matters is that it gives you a sense of hope and love, even in troubled times. Because, as we well know, life is many things but never straightforward.

Remember this: the body feels what the mind thinks. There is more to health than food and exercise. We thrive when we have a spiritual connection. Nurture your relationships and they will nurture you.

LEARNINGS

'Ageing is a matter of mind.
If you don't mind, it doesn't matter.'
—Author unknown

I started this book saying I wanted to follow in the footprints of those who'd gone before, in order to clear the path for those who come after. With that in mind, it seems only right that I should end the book with 80-year-old Tess. 'I'm becoming bolder, learning that every day is a gift,' she told me. 'We can do anything we like. We are wise. We are elders of excellence. We must love ourselves. We are OK … right now.'

Another thing Tess told me? 'I hate labels. Ignore the labels. They're limiting.'

So what have I learnt on this journey?

I have learnt that your life course is paramount. What goes before matters. The lifestyle you lead in your forties and fifties has a huge bearing on how well you'll be faring at 80. I'm trying to encourage my kids to think about that.

I have learnt that successful ageing is not an oxymoron and that engagement in life is the key to ageing well. We should be having more conversations about improving resilience in older age in the same way that we talk about increasing resilience in children and young adults. There is no such thing as 'too late' in life. We have the ability to change until the day we die.

I have learnt that a lot of it boils down to having a glass-half-full mentality. We rate our health, homes, relationships and material things against our own expectations – expectations that we construct ourselves. This subjective rating has a huge bearing on outcomes. We judge what we have against what we would like. Optimism is something we all need to practise. For some, it comes more naturally than for others, but the making of lemonade from life's lemons is a great philosophy to follow.

I have learnt that gratitude and forgiveness are profoundly protective in older age. Learn to forgive yourself and to forgive others. There is no room for bitterness in healthy ageing. The ability to play and create in retirement, and to cultivate younger friendships, will help you to age well. It is those simple things, rather than a whopping retirement income, that will make you happy. Now, I set aside time to stop and smell the roses, and immerse myself in the beauty of the world.

I have learnt that I need to prioritise my relationships with my loved ones above all else. These relationships are profoundly protective, especially as we age. They can be complicated and messy, and they require tolerance, attention and a sense of humour.

If you are lonely, it's not too late to develop new friendships or reconnect with friends who might have fallen aside along the way. Remember the past. Accept it, but don't dwell in it. Learn from the mistakes you've made, but try not to punish yourself or bury yourself in regret.

I have learnt that, as each year passes, I'm not on a downward slide into old age. I am optimistically hoping I have at least 20 good years ahead of me and I need to make them count. I know it's important to exercise daily and not put it on the back burner. I know that I will feel pain from time to time, as arthritis begins to bite and the natural ageing process takes hold, but that a positive mental attitude is vital in setting that to one side and moving forward.

I have learnt that dementia is not a given as we age. That I need to keep my brain active and challenged in the same way I need to keep my body active and challenged. To that end, I may well take up bridge, though right now Uno Flip with the grandchildren is about as complicated as it gets! I keep Sir Richard Faull's mantra top of mind: 'What's good for the heart is good for the head.'

I have learnt, too, that I have been blessed with a reasonably smooth transition into older age – but it doesn't happen that way for everyone, and it behoves the rest of us to consider those people who are struggling. It behoves us to care what happens to our fellow citizens. Are they well housed? Are we planning for a time when nearly half of over-65s will not own their homes? Do older people have ready access to the health system? Can they even get to a doctor, given they may not be able to drive and may live in remote areas? Are they receiving the appropriate care from government agencies charged with their welfare? I suspect the answer to all of those questions is no ... and if that is so, then we should all be lobbying decision-makers to better care for the needs of older people. Some older Kiwis are more disconnected and isolated than ever before, and the physical and mental toll is devastating. It's an unseen epidemic. At the risk of using what's become a slightly overused phrase, we need to be kind to each other, to really 'see' people in the community who may be alone and struggling, and then reach out to include them.

The New Zealand government does currently have a Healthy Ageing Strategy that presents 'the strategic direction for change and a set of actions to improve the health of older people, into and throughout their later years'. Its key themes are as follows:

1. Prevention, healthy ageing and resilience throughout people's older years.
2. Living well with long-term health conditions.
3. Improving rehabilitation and recovery from acute episodes.
4. Better support for older people with high and complex needs.
5. Respectful end-of-life care.

Strategies and goals are great to have, but they must be implemented. We need to hold governments to account on these goals, otherwise they're just empty words and unfulfilled promises.

* * *

As I finish this book, Chris and I are embarking on a new phase in our lives. We have decided to downsize, to simplify our lives. This has become remarkably freeing for both of us.

I remember how simple life used to be when we were younger, when it was just the two of us setting off into married life, when we had few trappings, few responsibilities and life held infinite promise ... Well, it feels a bit like that now.

Our children are grown and have lives and loves of their own. We're still extremely close to them, but we have shed a lot of that parental responsibility. We feel free to explore new interests, to learn new skills and to indulge new 'fads', as the family would call them. We're always trying new things: bringing old furniture to life with chalk paint (there was a time there when no wooden piece was safe!), learning to salsa (we discovered we had four left feet), becoming vegetarian (this happened after my interview with Gary Fraser from the Adventist Health Studies ... but I've lapsed since), paddleboarding, cycling and who knows what else? And we have a sense of purpose in our lives as our grandchildren continue to grow and flourish. We are so lucky to be able to play an active part in their lives.

This new life of ours has begun with a major declutter. No small task when you've lived in the same house for 45 years! We've spent hours poring over boxes full of photos and decades' worth of stuff loosely labelled 'memorabilia' that's stashed away in the attic. We may need to bring in a referee as we bicker away about what should stay and what should go, but all in all it is a remarkably liberating experience. All those things that seemed important in the 1970s, '80s and '90s have just merged into the minutiae of life. That is a benefit of age, I guess – the ability to look back and wonder why we managed to get ourselves into such a knot about things we now deem unimportant.

You know, there is a method to all this decluttering madness. Swedish sociology professor Lars Tornstam has a theory called 'gerotranscendence', in which he suggests we have the potential, as we enter old age, to move from a materialistic and rational point of view to a more altruistic and outward-looking one. Tornstam interviewed Swedish men and women between the ages of 52 and 97, and found that they had become more aware of previously hidden aspects of themselves, both good and bad.

They were more self-aware, more altruistic, less self-centred, and more inclined to rediscover their childhoods and relive happy memories.

In their relationships, they had become more selective and less superficial. They also spoke about an increasing need for solitude, time to themselves.

Their attitude to wealth had changed, and they had a greater awareness that possessions can ensnare and confine a person.

They found joy in challenging societal norms and appreciated the grey area to be found between right and wrong. They were more considered, more tolerant and broad-minded.

And, as far as cosmic insights went, they reported a sense that relatives who had died long ago were close by. They became interested in genealogy and discovering family trees.

Their fear of death receded, and they were increasingly curious about what might be next in store for them.

They also showed a renewed interest in nature and their connection to it, and delighted in the small things.

Tornstam's research shows that our minds continue to develop and change in older age. We have the ability to become more reflective, thoughtful, considerate and curious. In essence, we have the ability and the opportunity to put a lifetime's lessons to good use.

We are all guardians or kaitiaki of knowledge. Let's do our best to pass it on to future generations. Knowledge not only about our history, but also about the life lessons we have learnt along the way. We have blazed our own trail through the minefield of life, there are footprints to follow, and missteps to be avoided.

And so I return to the late Professor Morrie Schwartz, and a quote from his own book, *Morrie in His Own Words*: 'Keep your heart open for as long as you can, as wide as you can for others and especially for yourself. Be generous, decent and welcoming.'

FURTHER READING AND RESOURCES

1. Your Whole Being: Age Inside and Out

Rauch, Jonathan. *The Happiness Curve: Why Life Gets Better After Midlife*. London: Bloomsbury Publishing, 2018.

Sinclair, David A. *Lifespan: Why We Age – and Why We Don't Have To*. New York: Atria Books, 2019.

The University of Auckland. 'LiLACS NZ' (Life and Living in Advanced Age, a Cohort Study in New Zealand). https://www.fmhs.auckland.ac.nz/en/faculty/lilacs.html

Vaillant, George. *Aging Well: Surprising Guideposts to a Healthier Life*. New York: Little, Brown, 2002.

2. Thought for Food: Eating well

Blue Zones®. 'Food Guidelines'. https://www.bluezones.com/recipes/food-guidelines/

Hyman, Mark. *Young Forever: The Secrets to Living Your Longest, Healthiest Life*. London: Hodder & Stoughton, 2023.

Loma Linda University Health. 'Adventist Health Study-2'. https://adventisthealthstudy.org/studies/AHS-2

3. In Our Cups: Drinking

Alcohol Drug Helpline. 'Alcohol Drug Helpline homepage'. https://alcoholdrughelp.org.nz/ (Helpline: 0800 787 797)

Alcohol Healthwatch. 'Alcohol Healthwatch homepage'. https://www.ahw.org.nz/

Dann, Lotta. *Mrs D is going without: A Memoir*. Auckland: Allen & Unwin, 2014.

—*The Wine O'Clock Myth: The Truth You Need to Know about Women and Alcohol*. Auckland: Allen & Unwin, 2020.

Ministry of Health. 'Alcohol'. https://www.health.govt.nz/your-health/healthy-living/addictions/alcohol-and-drug-abuse/alcohol

Nasserzadeh, Sara. 'Episode 4: Drinking in Lockdown & Beyond with Professor Paul Wallace'. *the little black fish* podcast. https://podcasts.apple.com/us/podcast/drinking-in-lockdown-beyond-professor-paul-wallace/id1507622021?i=1000473306783

NZ Drug Foundation. 'Alcohol'. https://www.drugfoundation.org.nz/info/drug-index/alcohol/

4. Move It or Lose It: Exercise

Centers for Disease Control and Prevention. 'How much physical activity do older adults need?'. https://www.cdc.gov/physicalactivity/basics/older_adults/index.htm

Clear, James. *Atomic Habits: An Easy and Proven Way to Build Good Habits and Break Bad Ones*. London: Penguin Random House, 2018.

Harvard Health Publishing. 'Exercise and aging: Can you walk away from Father Time'. 9 March 2014. https://www.health.harvard.edu/staying-healthy/exercise-and-aging-can-you-walk-away-from-father-time

Valant, Jessica. 'Basic Pilates for Beginners – 15 Minute Pilates Workout'. Jessica Valant Pilates, YouTube, uploaded 18 September 2023. https://www.youtube.com/watch?v=_en_PIYjveg

5. The Great Obsession: Sleep

Espie, Colin. *Overcoming Insomnia: A Self-help Guide Using Cognitive Behavioural Techniques*. London: Little, Brown, 2021.

Foster, Russell. *Life Time: The New Science of the Body Clock, and How It Can Revolutionize Your Sleep and Health*. London: Penguin Books, 2022.

Gibson, Rosie. 'Sleep Support: A Sleep Handbook for Older People Living with Dementia.' Sleep–Wake Research Centre, Massey University, 2016. https://www.sleepwake.ac.nz/media/1134/sleep-support-revised-2017-inc-front.pdf

Loredo, Jose. 'Sleep and Aging'. University of California Television (UCTV), YouTube, uploaded 8 December2017. https://www.youtube.com/watch?v=OtbgWhzI7bU

6. Maintenance: Healthcare

Healthify He Puna Waiora. 'Ear care advice'. https://healthify.nz/hauora-wellbeing/e/ear-care-advice/

—'Eyes and Ageing'. https://healthify.nz/health-a-z/e/eyes-and-ageing/

—'Fungal nail infections'. https://healthify.nz/health-a-z/f/fungal-nail-infections/

—'Taking care of your teeth'. https://healthify.nz/health-a-z/o/oral-health-taking-care-of-your-teeth/

Melanoma New Zealand. 'Melanoma New Zealand homepage'. https://melanoma.org.nz/

7. The Long Goodbye: Dementia

Alzheimers New Zealand. 'Alzheimers New Zealand homepage'. https://alzheimers.org.nz/ (Helpline: 0800 004 001)

Burns, Jeffrey and Foundas, Anna. 'What's good for your heart is good for your brain'. Dana Foundation, YouTube, uploaded 14 July 2015. https://www.youtube.com/watch?v=vvJzdbHCDg0

Dementia New Zealand. 'Home Page | Dementia New Zealand'. https://dementia.nz/ (Helpline: 0800 444 776)

Faull, Richard. 'Rethinking the Brain: Richard Faull at TEDxAuckland'. TEDx Talks, YouTube, uploaded 2 September 2013. https://www.youtube.com/watch?v=NT_Z6kULoVw

Mitchell, Wendy. Somebody I Used to Know. London: Bloomsbury Publishing, 2018.

Snow, Teepa. 'Teepa Snow: Caring for Someone Who Has Dementia'. Teepa Snow's Positive Approach to Care, YouTube, uploaded 3 March 2020. https://www.youtube.com/watch?v=MA9s2vZflw4

—*Understanding the Changing Brain: Move from Surviving to Thriving with Teepa Snow's Tips and Insights*. Efland, North Carolina: Positive Approach to Care, 2021.

8. It Takes Two: Relationships

Age Concern. 'Loneliness research'. https://ageconcern.org.nz/Public/Info/Research/Loneliness_and_Social_Isolation_Research.aspx

Albom, Mitch. *Tuesdays with Morrie: an old man, a young man, and life's greatest lesson*. New York: Knopf Doubleday Publishing Group, 1997.

Massachusetts General Hospital and Harvard Medical School. Harvard Second Generation Study. 'Welcome to the Harvard Study of Adult Development'. https://www.adultdevelopmentstudy.org/

Office for Seniors/Te Tari Kaumātua. 'Eastern Bay Villages: Te Kokoru Manaakitanga'. Last modified 18 February 2022. https://officeforseniors.govt.nz/our-work/age-friendly-communities/2-age-friendly-case-studies/eastern-bay-case-study/

—'2022 Indicator: Enhancing opportunities for participation and social connection'. https://officeforseniors.govt.nz/assets/Uploads/Key-Area-4.-Enhancing-opportunities-for-participation-and-social-connection.pdf

Waldinger, Robert. 'Robert Waldinger: What makes a good life? Lessons from the longest study on happiness'. TED, YouTube, uploaded 26 January 2016. https://www.youtube.com/watch?v=8KkKuTCFvzI

—'The Secret to a Happy Life – Lessons from 8 Decades of Research | Robert Waldinger | TED'. TED, YouTube, uploaded 11 January 2023. https://www.youtube.com/watch?v=IStsehNAOL8

9. Grandparenting 101: Looking after kids

GrandFriends. 'GrandFriends'. https://www.grandfriends.nz/

Grandparents Raising Grandchildren. 'Grandparents Raising Grandchildren homepage'. https://www.grg.org.nz/

Parenting Place Charitable Trust. 'Parenting Place homepage'. https://parentingplace.nz/

Work and Income/Te Hiranga Tangata. 'Caring for someone else's child.' https://www.workandincome.govt.nz/eligibility/carers/care-someone-else-child.html

10. The R-word: Retirement

Hawes, Martin. *Twenty Good Summers: Work Less, Live More and Make the Most of your Money.* Sydney: Allen & Unwin, 2006.

Retirement Commission/Te Ara Ahunga Ora. 'Office of the Retirement Commissioner homepage'. https://retirement.govt.nz/

12. Dollars and Sense: Finances

Citizens Advice Bureau/Ngā Pou Whakawhirinaki o Aotearoa. 'Citizens Advice Bureau homepage'. https://www.cab.org.nz/

Eaqub, Shamubeel. 'Stories by Shamubeel Eaqub'. https://www.rnz.co.nz/authors/shamubeel-eaqub

Eldernet. 'Eldernet Knowledge Lab'. https://www.eldernet.co.nz/knowledge-lab

Financial Markets Authority/Te Mana Tatai Hokohoko. 'FMA: Consumer'. https://www.fma.govt.nz/consumer/

Holm, Mary. *Get Rich Slow: How to Grow Your Wealth the Safe and Savvy Way.* Auckland: Penguin, 2006.

—*Rich Enough?: A Laid-Back Guide for Every Kiwi*. Auckland: HarperCollins Publishers, 2018.

Massey University. 'New Zealand Retirement Expenditure Guidelines' report. First published September 2022. https://www.massey.ac.nz/documents/476/nz_retirement_expenditure_gudelines.pdf

MoneyTalks. 'MoneyTalks – Free budgeting help, debt help'. https://www.moneytalks.co.nz/ (Helpline: 0800 345 123)

Retirement Commission/Te Ara Ahunga Ora. 'Sorted – Your independent money guide'. https://sorted.org.nz/

—'Live Sorted – Retirement'. https://sorted.org.nz/guides/retirement

The Spinoff/Kiwibank. 'When the Facts Change, with Bernard Hickey' podcast. https://thespinoff.co.nz/podcasts/when-the-facts-change

13. Dotting i's and Crossing t's: Paperwork

Hawes, Martin. *Cracking Open the Nest Egg: How to Make your Retirement Savings Last the Distance*. Auckland: Upstart Press, 2021.

—*Family Trusts: The Must-have New Zealand Guide*. Auckland: Random House NZ, 2020.

MoneyHub. 'Prenuptial Agreements (Prenup) - The Definitive New Zealand Guide'. https://www.moneyhub.co.nz/prenuptial-agreements.html

Office for Seniors/Te Tari Kaumātua. 'Elder Abuse Response Service'. https://officeforseniors.govt.nz/our-work/raising-awareness-of-elder-abuse/elder-abuse-response-service/ (Helpline: 0800 EA NOT OK/0800 32 668 65)

Public Trust. 'Public Trust homepage'. https://www.publictrust.co.nz/ (Helpline: 0800 371 471)

The Retirement Villages Association of New Zealand (RVA). 'The Retirement Villages Association of New Zealand homepage'. https://www.retirementvillages.org.nz/

14. Not Buying Green Bananas!: Death

Blackhall, Leslie. 'Living, Dying and the Problem with Hope | Dr. Leslie Blackhall | TEDxCharlottesville'. TEDxTalks, YouTube, uploaded 12 January 2016. https://www.youtube.com/watch?v=KQEWc3LVfyc

Gibran, Khalil. *The Prophet*. London: William Heinemann, 1926.

Hillman, Ken. *A Good Life to the End: Taking Control of our Inevitable Journey through Ageing and Death*. Sydney: Allen & Unwin, 2017.

—'We're Doing Dying All Wrong | Ken Hillman | TEDxSydney'. TEDx Talks, YouTube, uploaded 15 June 2016. https://www.youtube.com/watch?v=gQVC-8WEB7s

Hospice New Zealand/Te Kahu Pairuri o Aotearoa. 'Hospice New Zealand homepage'. https://www.hospice.org.nz/

Organ Donation New Zealand. 'Organ Donation New Zealand homepage'. https://donor.co.nz/

15. Heartache: Grief

Brown, Brené. 'David Kessler on Grief and *Finding Meaning*'. *Unlocking Us* podcast, released 31 March 2020. https://brenebrown.com/podcast/david-kessler-and-brene-on-grief-and-finding-meaning/

Frankl, Victor E. *Man's Search for Meaning.* London: Penguin, 1959.

Grief Centre. 'Grief Centre homepage'. https://www.griefcentre.org.nz/

Hone, Lucy. *Resilient Grieving: Finding Strength and Embracing Life After a Loss That Changes Everything.* Auckland: Allen & Unwin, 2017.

Kessler, David. *Finding Meaning: The Sixth Stage of Grief.* New York: Scribner, 2020.

16: Riding the Wave: Resilience

Anxiety NZ. 'Anxiety NZ homepage'. https://anxiety.org.nz/ (Helpline: 0800 ANXIETY/0800 269 438)

Emmons, Robert A. *Thanks!: How Practising Gratitude Can Make You Happier.* New York: Houghton Mifflin, 2008.

Health Promotion Agency. 'Home | Depression and Anxiety'. https://www.depression.org.nz/ (Helpline: 0800 111 757)

Learnings

Ministry of Health/Manatū Hauora. 'Healthy Ageing Strategy'. Published online 13 December 2016. https://www.health.govt.nz/publication/healthy-ageing-strategy

Tornstam, Lars. *Gerotranscendence: A Developmental Theory of Positive Aging.* New York: Springer Publishing Company, 2005.

Schwartz, Morrie. *Morrie In His Own Words: Life Wisdom from a Remarkable Man.* London: Pan Books, 2005.

ACKNOWLEDGMENTS

My thanks to the HarperCollins team for their oversight and encouragement, especially to Holly Hunter and Kimberley Davis in New Zealand, and Rachel Dennis in Australia.

So many academics and medical people have helped me with this book. Special thanks to Professor Ngaire Kerse, Dr Hamish Jamieson, Emeritus Professor Dame Peggy Koopman-Boyden, Dr Gary Fraser of the Adventist Health Studies, Dr Rosie Gibson, Dr Vanessa Burtholt, Dr Louise Parr Brownlie, Dr Chris Stephens, Dr Xaviour Walker, and all those who've contributed to the extraordinary Harvard Study of Adult Development. Thank you for your knowledge and your commitment to finding better ways for older people to age.

The thanks of an entire nation should go to Professor Sir Richard Faull and his team at Auckland's Centre for Brain Research for their work on neurodegenerative diseases of the brain, a tiny portion of which I have mined for this book.

The Brainwave Trust Aotearoa has given me invaluable knowledge about early brain development and the critical importance of relationships for the developing brain.

Thank you to Age Concern's former CEO Stephanie Clear; New Zealand's Retirement Commissioner, Jane Wrightson; Mary Holm and Rhonda Powell for being so generous with their time.

My thanks, too, to Johann van den Berg, Nola Forsyth and Coralie Gibson of the Grief Centre for their considered input, to Skylight for access to their wonderful resources, and to my friend Gilly Tyler for talking so freely about her own grief.

I am so grateful to the many older people who have been so candid in sharing their thoughts about their ageing journey.

And finally, to my husband, Chris – thank you for standing beside me this past fifty-plus years. Your support and encouragement mean the world.